Host
Defense
and
Infection

M. T. Labro, MD, PhD

Hoechst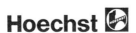

Marcel Dekker, Inc.   **New York•Basel•Hong Kong**

ISBN: 0-8247-9218-1

The publisher offers discounts on this book when ordered in bulk quantities. For more information, write to Special Sales/Professional Marketing at the address below.

This book is printed on acid-free paper.

MARCEL DEKKER, INC.
270 Madison Avenue, New York, New York 10016

Current printing (last digit):
10 9 8 7 6 5 4 3 2 1

PRINTED IN THE UNITED STATES OF AMERICA

CONTENTS

INTRODUCTION

The evolutionary process has culminated in a highly sophisticated human immune defense system. It is now clear that this system is involved not only in recognition and elimination of "nonself" cells and molecules, but also in homeostasis; however, its main role is in the defenses of host integrity against the environment and malignancies. The basic concept emerged from the scientific revolution of the late 19th century with the discovery of microbial pathogenicity and the main components of the host defense system (antibodies, complement and phagocytes). The pioneers in the field of immunology opened the way for scientists in the 20th century who, with the help of technology, have engendered an "explosion" of fundamental knowledge. The host defense system is now known to involve multiple cell subpopulations regulated by pleiotropic overlapping messengers (cytokines) and cell–cell interactions mediated by cell-adhesion molecules (C-AMs) and other receptors.

Discoveries of new mediators, new functions and new concepts daily modify the moving picture of immunology, and make it difficult for the nonspecialists to apprehend. However, a knowledge of basic immunological responses is essential to optimize treatment of diseases, particularly those due to microorganisms.

This short review presents in a somewhat simplified manner the main actors, their role in defense against microorganisms and how anti-infectious agents modulate the various effectors involved.

Man, Microorganisms and Science: An Ongoing Story (Figure 1)

As in all fields of science, our understanding of the interactions between man and microorganisms is not the result of a continuum of findings but of step-by-step discoveries. The first step was the definition of human bodily structure ("Anatomy Era," up to the 16th century). The "Cellular Era" began with the discovery of the microscope (17th century), which enabled T. Swann (early 19th century) to establish the cellular nature of plants and animals. A. Van Leuwenhoek's invention opened the doors to microbiology but the major advances were based on the critical findings of pathogenicity and virulence by Pasteur, Koch and others in the 19th century. At the same time, the "Immunology Era" began when Metchnikoff, Behring, Bordet, Ehrlich, and others brought to light some of the crucial components of natural defense systems. Finally, therapy against infectious diseases, mainly an empirical process until the 19th century, has seen prophylactic regimens (asepsis and vaccination) develop parallel to our understanding of pathogenicity. The discovery of the first anti-infectious agents in the 19th century was followed by the revolution of the mid 20th century, when the first antibiotics were successfully introduced into the therapeutic armamentarium. Now, on the threshold of the third millennium, new strategies are required to counter the growing resistance of most microorganisms to these therapeutic weapons. In particular, the aim is to restore (and/or enhance) the natural defense system to face microbial aggression. These approaches include the use of immune modulators (bacterial, fungal products, colony stimulating factors [CSFs]) and gene therapy. One existing possibility is to associate host defense enhancement with antimicrobial agents. Synergistic combinations of immune modulators (in particular CSFs) and classical antibiotics are already assessed in experimental models of infection, while at least one "immunomodulating antibiotic" has already been developed.

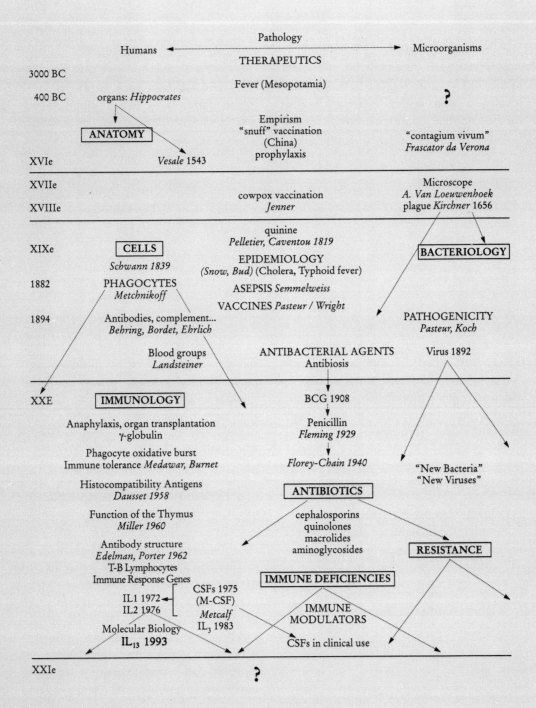

Figure 1 Men, microorganisms and science.

I

BASIC KNOWLEDGE OF HOST DEFENSES AGAINST INFECTION

Multicellular organisms find themselves surrounded by single-cell (and "precellular") microbes, only some of which are pathogenic. Phylogenic evolution has selected several features that protect the host from aggressive intruders (Figure 2):

1. Natural barriers (external protection)

2. Innate defense mechanisms, of which the phagocytes are the most important, phylogenetically ubiquitous effectors

3. Specific immune mechanisms, which form an elaborate defense system with highly specialized weapons directed against specific invaders

Human beings and mammals, at the top of the phylogenetic tree, possess these three levels of defense, and they are potent enough to protect them from most pathogens (it has been evaluated that during a human lifetime, a total of 150 pathogenic encounters result in fewer than 10 infections).

At the end of the late 20th century, the growing numbers of immunocompromised individuals, partly a consequence of therapeutic progress, is more that ever placing the spotlight on the natural anti-infectious system, which is schematized in Figure 3.

I. Innate Versus Acquired Immunity

"Innate immunity" refers to natural resistance to infection regardless of the pathogen and is immediately triggered when the protective barriers are breached. In contrast, "specific immunity" takes days to become effective while the antigenic message is being deciphered and specific weapons are being developed.

A. Innate Immunity

The nonspecific antimicrobial systems involve both cellular and humoral effectors.

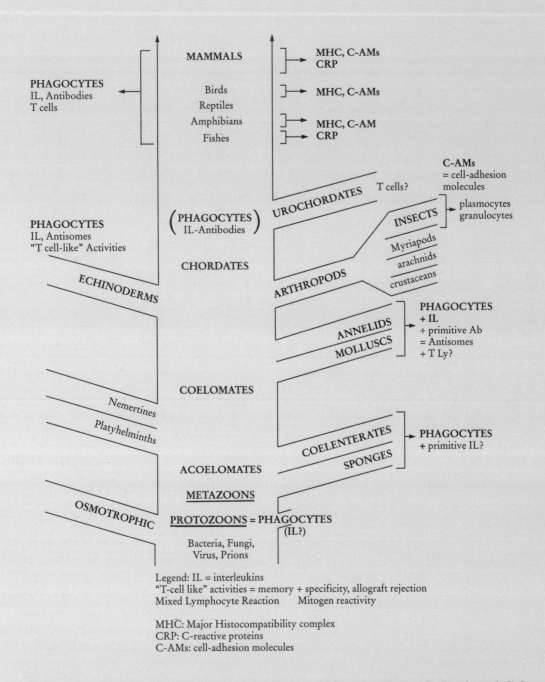

Figure 2 The phylogenetic tree of immune defenses. (From G. Beck and G.S. Habicht: Immunol. Today 1991, 12, 180-183, and Marchalonis J., Schluter S. F.: Scand. J. Immunol. 1990, 32, 13-20).

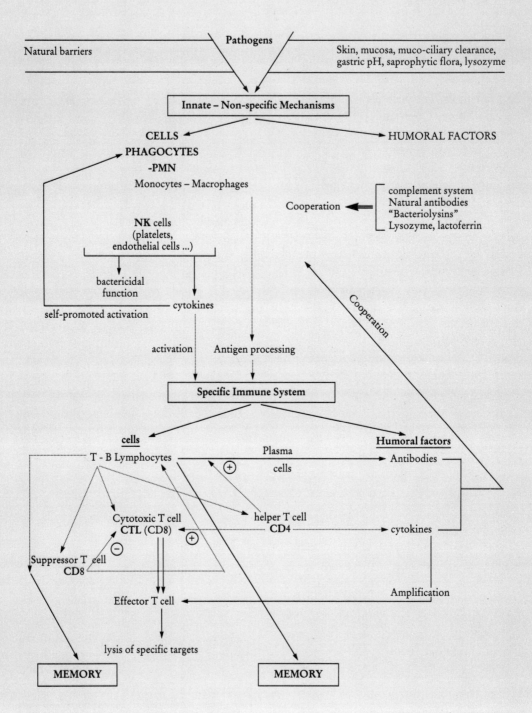

Figure 3   Anti-infectious defenses.

1. Phagocytes

a. Introduction: Definition

In the late 19th century, Metchnikoff recognized phagocytosis as a crucial mechanism in antibacterial defense. At the same time, Conheim, Helmholz and others outlined the role of phagocytes in the inflammatory reaction. Since that time, much has been learned about phagocytes, which still appear as the cornerstone of antimicrobial defenses.

The term "professional phagocytes" covers cells whose main functions are engulfing and destroying foreign materials. They all derive from a bone marrow progenitor (pluripotent stem cell) forming the myelomonocytic lineage (Figure 4). Mature effector cells are polymorphonuclear neutrophils (PMNs), blood monocytes and tissue-derived macrophages. Phagocytes use the same mechanisms to eradicate microorganisms, although PMNs appear to be the more potent and, contrary to macrophages which can be a "safe haven" for facultative/obligate intracellular pathogens, PMNs do not permit intracellular multiplication, with the exception of some *Ehrlichia* species. Platelets and endothelial cells have recently been evidenced as bactericidal against some pathogens (in particular *Trypanosoma*). However, the main role of these cells in immediate defenses appears to be the release of mediators activating phagocytes and leading to their selective attraction to the inflammatory focus.

b. Phagocytic Destruction of Pathogens (Figure 5)

As soon as microorganisms have penetrated into tissues, a *localized inflammatory reaction* is generated by their interaction with resident macrophages, mastocytes and humoral factors. This results first in dilatation of capillaries and increased permeability, with subsequent extravasation of serum constituents, particularly complement-system proteins. Activation of complement leads to generation of chemotactic factors (mainly C5a). Microorganisms may also release chemotaxins. Both kinds of signal, as well as some cytokines (e.g., IL-8), create a chemoattractant gradient within the tissue. At the same time, the inflammatory response induces modifications of local endothelial cells and platelets (expression of new receptors, release of mediators) that permit strong adhesion of marginated PMNs. PMNs then enter the tissues by diapedesis and, guided by the chemotactic gradient, migrate to the infected site (*chemotaxis*). The next step is in adhesion to the invaders, which is favoured by opsonization (deposit of complement split products C3b and inactivated C3b—and/or immunoglobulins). These opsonins are recognized by specific receptors on PMN membranes and permit strong association of PMN to bacteria. Binding can also involve carbohydrate recognition (lectin-mediated phagocytosis). Following adhesion, bacteria are engulfed within the vacuole (*phagosome*); activation of the PMNs leads to the assembly of a complex enzyme system (NADPH oxidase) located on the membrane of the phagosome, and the generation of strong oxidative species (superoxide anion, O_2^-.). Fusion of PMN granules to the phagosome (now a *phagolysosome*) exposes the engulfed bacteria to various lytic mechanisms classified into two groups: oxygen-dependent mechanisms (transformation of O_2^-. into more potent reactive oxygen species by the myeloperoxidase [MPO] system released from azurophilic granules) and oxygen-independent mechanisms (lysozyme, antibiotic peptides-defensins and proteins). A simplified scheme of these two kinds of mechanism is shown in Figure 6.

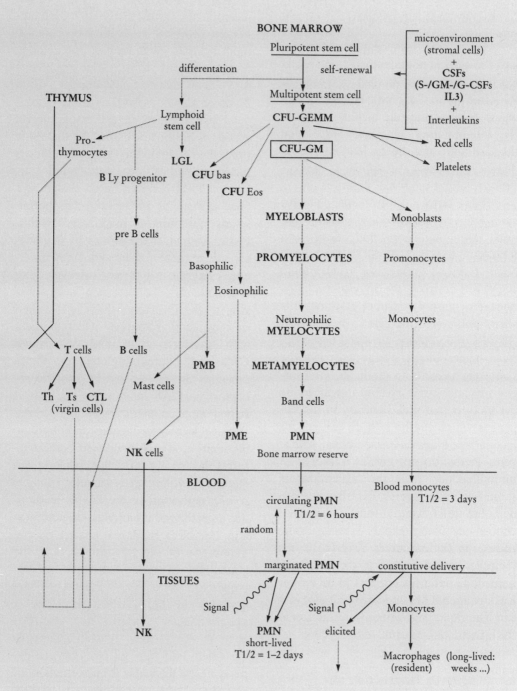

Figure 4 Origin and fate of effector cells in the natural defense.

After killing, digestion of microorganisms is performed by a panoply of hydrolytic enzymes released from the granules.

Monocytes and macrophages display similar bactericidal activity except for their delayed response in hours compared to minutes for PMNs after the inflammatory signals — and the oxygen-dependent killing systems: monocytes possess significantly less MPO than PMN, and macrophages are completely devoid of this enzyme. The late phases of oxidant generation thus do not occur in their phagolysosomes; this may explain the somewhat lower cidal activity for many bacterial and fungal species.

Destruction of bacteria may also occur in the external medium. Similarly, PMNs and other phagocytes can kill virus-infected or tumor cells after adhesion to their targets and release of oxidants and other lytic substances into the intercellular space.

c. Inflammation

For the complete process to occur, phagocytes have to be fully activated by optimal concentrations of opsonized or nonopsonized microorganisms. However, before contact with their targets induces activation, they are prepared by other signals involved in adhesion to the endothelium and chemotaxis; this "pre-activated" state is termed "priming." If the signals are overabundant, phagocytes may be activated before reaching their designated targets and release their destructive compounds (enzymes and oxidants) in the surrounding tissues, with subsequent cell and tissue damage; this is a key mechanism in the excessive inflammatory reaction often associated with infectious diseases. The production of cytokines, in particular TNF, is also thought to play a direct role in tissue damage or to further enhance phagocyte-induced damage.

d. Other Functions of Phagocytes

In addition to their destructive activity for foreign materials (and sometimes unfortunately, for host tissues), phagocytes have other functions that are part of the general anti-infectious process:

The synthesis and release of various cytokines that may potentiate their own function (autocrine regulation) or modify the activity of other cells (this subject will be dealt with after the general presentation of the effectors involved in host defense, since the cytokine network is a model of intercellular regulation).

The synthesis and production of other proteins that up-regulate some of their activities (in particular, various heat shock proteins, actin, fibronectin, opsonin receptors).

The production of various regulatory molecules (leucotrienes and prostaglandins derived from arachidonic acid via the lipoxygenase and cyclooxygenase pathways, phagocytosis-activating factors, steroid hormones, coagulation factors and complement components, endorphins, etc.).

Debridement and wound healing. Both macrophages and PMNs act to remodel sites of injury by the secretion of proteolytic enzymes and by endocytosis and intracellular degradation of the extracellular matrix and cellular debris. Furthermore, macrophage secretion of angiogenic molecules, e.g. TGF-α, bombesin and nerve growth factor on the one hand and phagocyte synthesis of extracellular matrix components (fibronectin, chondroitin sulfate, heparan-sulfate, proteogly-

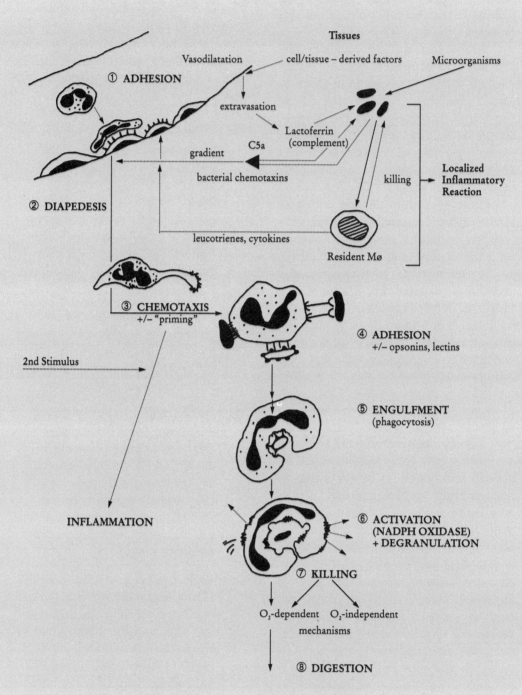

Figure 5   Main steps of phagocyte (PMN) activity.

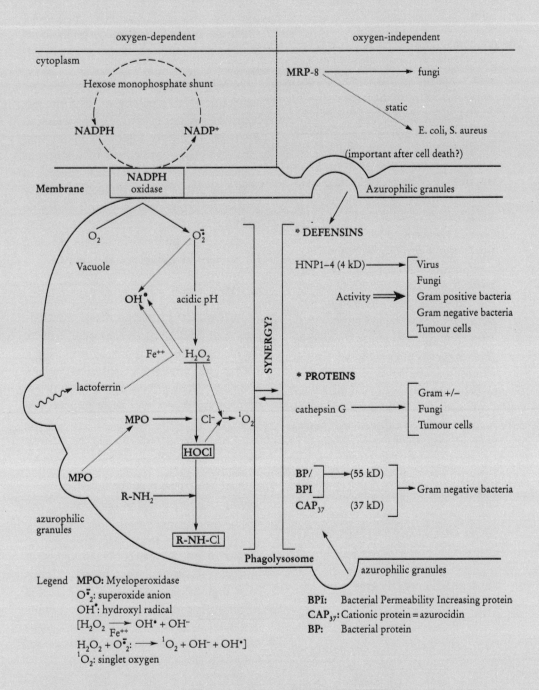

Figure 6 Mechanisms of PMN-mediated bacterial killing.

can, etc.) on the other are probably involved in the repair of altered tissues.

The synthesis of nitric oxide (NO) following immunological activation and induction of nitric oxide synthase. This compound, generated from L-arginine in the presence of NADPH, is cytostatic/cytotoxic for microorganisms (in particular fungi, helminths and protozoa) and tumor cells. The role of this pathway as an effector mechanism in macrophage cytotoxicity has now been demonstrated for a number of microorganisms (*Cryptococcus neoformans, Corynebacterium parvum, Toxoplasma gondii, Leishmania major* and *Mycobacterium avium*). The biological significance of NO production by neutrophils remains to be elucidated.

Finally, a major role of macrophages is their participation in the elaboration of specific defenses since they play a major role in *antigen-processing and presentation* to T lymphocytes, in association with class I or II major histocompatibility complex (MHC) molecules, depending on the T cell subset.

2. Other Cell Effectors Involved in Nonspecific Immune Defenses

a. Natural Killer (NK) and Lymphocyte Activated Killer (LAK) Cells

NK cells are a discrete subset of lymphocytes distinct from B and T cells, which lack antigen-recognition molecules (T cell receptor [TCR]) and surface immunoglobulins. LAK cells are a subset of NK which, upon activation by lymphokines (interleukin-2 [IL-2]), are able to kill several target cells. They derive from the lymphoid stem cell in the bone marrow, mostly have the large granular lymphocyte morphology, but kill a variety of target cells in a MHC-non-restricted fashion. NK cells have functions other than simple spontaneous cytotoxicity and regulate several cell types.

NK cells appear to kill by the same mechanisms as phagocytes, with the exception of phagocytosis, i.e.: adhesion to the target (tumor or infected cells); effector cell activation; release of toxic substances in the intercellular space, in particular nonoxidant molecules (serine proteases, granzymes A-G and TNF-like activity); detachment and recycling. The cytotoxic mechanisms of phagocytes and killer cells are compared in Table 1.

b. Mast Cells

Mast cells derived from multipotent stem cells play an important role in the inflammatory reaction by secreting a variety of mediators. Undifferentiated precursors in the bone marrow migrate to various tissues and differentiate into two types of mast cells:

Mucosal mast cells

Connective tissue type mast cells (containing large amounts of histamine)

In addition, these cells also play an important role in allergic (IgE-mediated) immune reactions. Mature mast cells have high-affinity receptors for IgE and binding triggers the release of histamine and other mediators which, in turn, leads to localized or generalized allergic reactions (e.g., anaphylaxis).

3. Humoral Factors: The Complement System (Figure 7)

Complement comprises a set of proteins that work to eliminate microorganisms and other antigens from tissues and blood. This task is achieved either

Table 1 Cytotoxic Mechanisms of Cellular Effectors

Cell	Origin	Receptors	Granules	Cytotoxicity
PMN	CFU-G (bone marrow)	FcR_I (inducible) FcR_{II} FcR_{III} CR_I β_2 integrins CR_3 $CR_4(+)$	Azurophilic + specific + others? (tertiary gr.)	Not spontaneous (+ stimulus) ±Phagocytosis O_2-dependent + O_2-independent ADCC+
Monocytes ↓ Macrophages	CFU-M (bone marrow)	FcR_I (constitutive) FcR_{II} β_2 integrins CR_3 CR_4	+	Not spontaneous ±Phagocytosis O_2-dependent (<PMN; MPO↓) + O_2-independent ADCC+
NK cells ↓cytokines LAK cells	LGL (bone marrow) Macrophage + (IL_2+M-CSF)	FcR_{III} β_2 integrins CR_3 $CR_4(+)$	Azurophilic	Spontaneous No phagocytosis (some exceptions!) O_2-independent (granzymes, TNF-like proteins) ADCC+
CTL (CD8T cells) (Some CD4T cell subsets)	Lymphoid stem cell ↓ Thymus differentiation	TCR-CD_3 LFA_1 CR_3 CR_4	+	Antigen-specific (MHC class I restricted) No phagocytosis O_2-independent (lymphotoxin perforin)

FcR, receptor for immunoglobulin Fc; CR, complement receptors (see Table 2); ADCC, antibody-dependent cytotoxicity; TCR, T cell receptor; LFA, lymphocyte function–associated antigens.

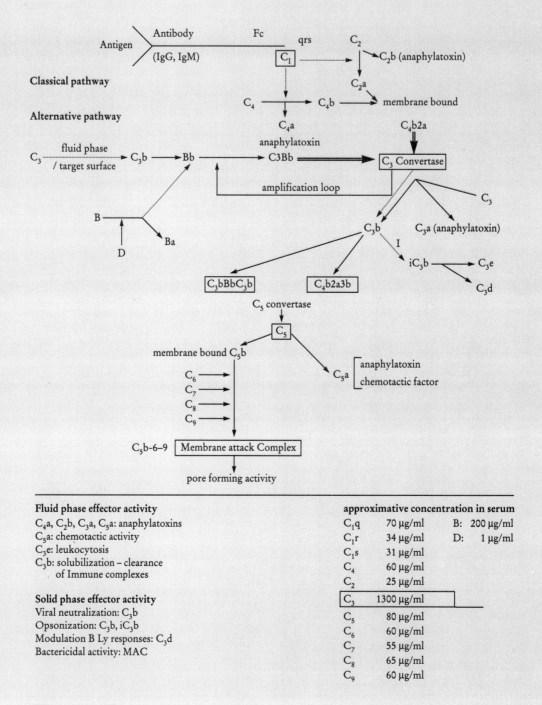

Figure 7 The complement system.

by complement alone or by complement components cooperating with antibodies and/or cells expressing complement receptors.

At least 90% of plasma complement is synthesized by the liver. Cytokine mediators of the acute-phase response (IL-6, TNF) and dexamethasone may increase this hepatic synthesis two- to fivefold. Complement synthesis by tissue monocytes and macrophages probably plays an important role in local complement-mediated host defense. This synthesis is modulated by gamma-interferon and LPS.

The complement system involves nearly 30 plasma and membrane proteins. It consists of two activation pathways, a single terminal pathway, regulatory proteins and complement receptors.

Activation of the classical pathway is triggered by the binding of C1 (a trimolecular complex of C1q, C1r and C1s) to the Fc portion of antibodies (IgG or IgM) associated with their specific antigens. Activated C1s cleaves C4 into C4a and C4b and C2 and C2a and C2b. C2a binds noncovalently to C4b, which itself is bound to the target particle, to form C4b2a C3 convertase.

The other activation pathway (alternative pathway) can function in the absence of antibodies and is basically spontaneous; it appears as the phylogenetically most ancient system. It is initiated by the binding of C3 to host or foreign surfaces and hydrolysis of the intramolecular thioester bond of C3 either in the fluid phase or at the cell surface, leading to conformational changes in C3 (to a C3b or C3b-like conformation). The C3b-like molecule reacts with factors B and D to form a surface-bound C3b-Bb convertase. The two C3 convertases (C4b 2a and C3b Bb) are homologous and generate multiple molecules of C3b. C3b can later be inactivated (iC3b).

Both C3b and iC3b are potent opsonins; when complement activation continues, C5 convertase (C4b 2a 3b or C3b Bb 3b) splits C5 into C5a (chemotactic) and C5b (membrane-bound). The terminal pathway is the sequential addition of C6 to C8 and multiple C9 (up to 18) molecules. The complex formed with C5b and C9 (membrane attack complex [MAC]) leads to membrane destruction by pore-formation mechanisms.

Regulatory proteins include inhibitors that prevent spontaneous activation in the fluid phase, regulators that dampen or enhance the normal action against targets, and inhibitors that protect host cells from the destructive action of complement.

Complement receptors are expressed on a variety of cell types that handle microorganisms and antigens. They permit recognition of opsonized targets, transduction of signals within cell and induction of cellular responses (such as phagocytosis and chemotaxis). Phagocytic cells express CR1, CR2 and C5a receptors (Table 2).

B. Specific Immunity

1. Introduction

The specific immune system must distinguish "self" from "non-self." This distinction is made by an elaborate specific-recognition system involving essentially T and B lymphocytes. The existence of the two major lymphocyte subsets that serve distinct functions in the generation of immune responses was first appreciated in 1958 by Mitchell and Miller: T cells being involved in delayed-type hypersensitivity, cytotoxicity and regulation, and B cells being responsible for antibody production. The subdivision of both classes was defined later, in particular, with the identification of T

Table 2 Complement Receptors and Host Defense

Name	Ligand	Cell	Functions
C5aR	C5a C5a des Arg	PMN Monocytes Mast cells	Margination Chemotaxis
C3aR C4aR	C3a C4a	PMN (+) Eosinophils Monocytes	
CR1	C3b>C4b>iC3b	PMN, monocytes Macrophages (+) B cells Eosinophils T cell subset (+)	Adhesion Phagocytosis Activation
CR3	iC3b, LPS β-glucan, fibrinogen	Monocytes, PMN Tissue macro- phages (+) Cytotoxic T cells NK cells Eosinophils	Adhesion Phagocytosis Activation
CR4	iC3b, endothelial cells	Monocytes (+) PMN (+) Cytotoxic T cells Tissue macro- phages NK cells Eosinophils (+)	Adhesion Phagocytosis Activation
CR2	C3d, gp350 Epstein-Barr virus	B lymphocytes	Modulation of responses? Virus entry

helper, T suppressor/cytotoxic lymphocytes. Other subsets are now defined on the basis of immunological markers and/or lymphokines production and/or specialized function.

T and B lymphocyte progenitors derive from the same multipotent hematopoietic stem cell in the bone marrow that gives rise to progenitors of other hematopoietic lineages. The maturational progression along the B and T differentiation pathway takes place either in the bone marrow (B cell lineage) or in the thymus (T cell lineage). As for the hematopoietic lineages, environmental factors (stromal cells and a variety of soluble molecules) regulate the maturation process.

Lymphocyte traffic and homing into peripheral lymphoid tissues is a prerequisite for the immune system to fulfill its function of immune surveillance. T and B cells home preferentially in distinct lymphoid compartments and some adhesion molecules (known as "homing receptors") regulate lymphocyte–endothelial interactions.

2. Repartition of T and B Lymphocytes in Lymphoid Organs

T cells comprise approximately 100% of thymus lymphocytes, 80% of peripheral blood lymphocytes, 60% of lymph node lymphocytes, 45% of spleen lymphocyte and only 10% of bone marrow lymphocytes. Conversely, B cells represent the main lymphocyte population in the bone marrow and are also concentrated into the spleen, an important site of antibody production. Other localizations of importance for the immune response are the gut-and bronchus-associated lymphoid tissues (two sites important for IgA production) and the skin-associated lymphoid tissue.

Peripheral T cells live for years. Clonal expansion may occur regionally after local antigenic stimulation but due to T cell recirculation, the entire body becomes susceptible to re-challenge. B cells do not live as long as T cells, but are equally mobile.

a. T Lymphocyte Biology

T Cell Receptor and Antigen Recognition

Thymus-derived lymphocytes (T cells) possess critical functions in the immune response. They are able to function as regulatory and effector cells and to carry immunologic memory. They are clonally restricted, which means that each T cell can recognize and become activated by one (or a closely related, "cross-reactive") antigen. This specificity is dependent on the T cell receptor (TCR), a two-chain (α-β), disulfide-linked heterodimer that shares similarities to immunoglobulin structure. This TCR recognizes antigens only when they are associated with MHC class I molecules (HLA-A-, -B, -C) for cytotoxic T cells and with MHC class II molecules (HLA-DR) for helper T cells. Indeed, the correct functioning of TCR is dependent upon the CD3 complex, five additional integral membrane proteins, noncovalently associated with TCR (Ti) which regulates assembly and expression of the receptor and is responsible for transmembrane traduction of signals following ligand binding to Ti.

Antigen-presenting cells (APCs) belong mainly to the mononuclear phagocyte system. However, other types of cells (endothelial and glial cells, primed B cells) may act as APCs.

Antigen handling by APC is not yet well understood; it involves:

1. Antigen acquisition by APCs

2. Structural modification of antigen to allow association with MHC

3. Transport of processed materials to cell surface

The major gateway into the class II pathway is the endosomal compartment where bacteria reside primarily. When bacteria evade into cytoplasm (and for soluble proteins introduced into the cytosol), peptides derived from proteolysis translocate to the endoplasmic reticulum, where they bind to MHC class I molecules and later become associated to the cell surface. It must be stressed that MHC class I molecules are expressed on virtually all cells whereas few express class II molecules (APC, B lymphocytes). MHC class II products may be induced by IFN-γ on endothelial and epithelial cells and fibroblasts.

Apart from the MHC (class I/II) binding ligand to the TCR, another specific ligand exists on APCs, the B7/BBI molecule, which seems to regulate lymphokine production by T cells via a receptor designated as CD28. Another T cell molecule involved in activation (or to maintain activation) is the CD45 molecule, which exists in many isoforms in various T cell subsets.

T Cell Subsets

T cell subsets are defined according to their specific functions and often by surface markers reacting with monoclonal antibodies.

Effector T Cells

1. Cytotoxic T lymphocytes recognize antigens associated with class I MHC products on the presenting cell (which results in generation of "primed" cytotoxic T cells) and on target cells (e.g., virus-infected or tumor cells), which they can lyse by the mean of cytotoxic molecules (perforin, TNF-like molecules, etc.). Cytotoxic T cells possess the CD8 marker.

2. Delayed-typed hypersensitivity T cells are responsible for DTH reactions. They recognize antigens associated with class II MHC products and possess the CD4 marker. Their proinflammatory activity is supported by the production of IL-2.

Regulator T Cells

Two kinds of T cells control the development of effector T and B lymphocytes: the first one is helper T cells (TH). They are CD4-positive, produce IL-2 in vitro after activation and enhance (or permit) B and T cell effector function, in particular antibody productions. Recently, different subsets of helper T cells have been defined according to lymphokine production. TH1 cells produce IL-2, IL-3, TNF, IFN-γ and GM-CSF, and support differentiation of activated B cells that secrete IgM, IgG2a and IgG3 (see below), whereas TH2 cells produce IL-4, IL-5, IL-10, IL-3, GM-CSF and TNF, support proliferation of quiescent B cells and differentiation into IgM-, IgG1-, and IgG3-secreting cells. Conversely, T suppressor cells (TS), which are CD8-positive, negatively regulate immune responses. They probably also play an important role in acquired immunologic tolerance. The immunologic memory seems to be a property of a TCD4 subset different from that of helper T cells.

b. **B Lymphocyte Biology**

Bone marrow-derived lymphocytes are responsible for antibody production.

Antibodies

The role of antibodies in natural

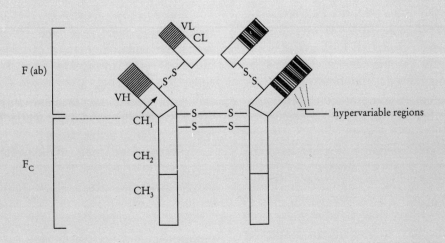

Figure 8 Immunoglobulin structure.

defenses was proposed at the end of the 19th century. Their chemical structure was first elucidated by Porter and Edelman in the mid 20th century. They belong to the immunoglobulin (Ig) family and are produced by B cell—derived plasmocytes. There are three major classes of Ig that possess structural similarities (Figure 8). They are heterodimers of heavy (H) and light (L) polypeptide chains linked by disulfide bridges. The N-terminal regions of H and L chains are the variable parts of the antibody, differing from one antibody to another and thus permitting the binding to one specific antigen. This part is designated as F(ab) (a fragment for antigen-binding). The C-terminal end of the molecule has a constant structure for each Ig class and subclass and confers various biologic functions. It is called Fc (a fragment that crystallizes).

Ig Classes and Subclasses
(Table 3)

Light chains exist in two classes, kappa and lambda (K and Λ); heavy chains exist as five classes (isotypes): gamma, alpha, mu, delta and epsilon for IgG, IgA, IgM, IgD and IgE. Each heavy chain associates with the same light chain in a single Ig. IgGs are the most abundant serum Ig. By crossing the placental barrier, they are the only antibodies to provide passive immunity to the newborn up to 3-6 months (half-life 21 days). Four subclasses are defined (IgG1, IgG2, IgG3, IgG4) which display some biologic differences (in particular for opsonization and complement activation).

IgAs are present at low concentration in the serum but they are the main Igs in the secretory antibody system and provide antimicrobial protection at various mucosal sites. Secretory IgA, in particular in the gastrointestinal tract, have a special configuration (two IgA molecules associated with a polypeptide chain—secretory piece) that confers resistance to proteolytic digestion. There are two subclasses, IgA1 and 2.

IgM (macroglobulin) is composed of five IgM subunits arranged in a pinwheel-like array, with the Fc portions in the center held together by joining chains.

IgEs are the classic skin-sensitizing, anaphylactic antibodies; their biologic properties depend on their high-affinity binding to specific receptors on mast cells and basophils.

Right now the biologic role of the IgD is not clearly understood.

B Cells

The best differentiation marker is Ig itself, whose nature changes following maturation.

Primitive B cell precursors have μ chains in their cytoplasm and no surface Ig. Then, intact cytoplasmic and membrane IgM are detected. Mature B cells possess surface IgM only as well as IgD (the function of which is still unclear). B cell activation results in division maturation into plasma cells that are the antibody-secreting cells. This activation may or may not depend on T cell triggering.

For the majority of antigens, TH cells, specifically primed, and their secretory products (lymphokines) are essential to trigger B cells to mature into plasma cells. This process also involves "Ig switching," since the first antibody response is of the IgM type while later IgG, A or E may be produced.

Some antigens, e.g., polysaccharide polymers, may trigger B cells directly; they mainly provoke a slight IgM response.

Summary

Both B and T lymphocytes identify antigens by recirculating through lymphoid tissues. The key recognition events are mediated by two signals delivered to lymphocytes: the first signal is provided by the binding of the lymphocyte antigen receptor to specialized APCs; this binding leads to the delivery of a second set of signals, required for lymphocyte proliferation and differentiation (for instance, binding of B7/BBI to CD28 and

Table 3 Subclasses of Ig

	Mean adult serum concentration (g/L)	Properties	
		Complement Fixation	Placental transfer
Total IgG	11.5 ± 3.0		
IgG1	6.0 ± 2.0	++	+
IgG2	3.0 ± 1.8	+	+
IgG3	0.4 ± 0.14	+++	+
IgG4	0.2 ± 0.16	-	+
IgM	1.0 ± 0.25	+++	-
IgA	2.0 ± 0.60	-	-
IgD	0.030	-	-
IgE	<0.001	-	-

participation of CD3, CD45 for initiation and/or maintainance of the response, e.g., IL-2 and other lymphokine production).

The initiation of immune responses depends critically on the recirculation of lymphocytes and delivery of effector cells to their site of action. CTLs must home to sites of intracellular infection, TH cells to germinal centers of lymph nodes and B cells to various locations (depending on the class of antibody they secrete).

Then the effector phase of the immune response takes place (for instance, destruction of infected targets by CTLs and macrophage activation by TH 1 cells).

Finally, establishment of cell memory, a critical event in vaccination, is associated with changes in number and state of differentiation of the cells. The steps involved in the specific immune response are schematized in Figures 9-11.

γδ *T Lymphocytes*

The discovery of a new subset of lymphocytes according to the nature of the TCR, now known as γδ T cells, has triggered much speculation as to their possible biologic functions. Like the more numerous αß T lymphocytes, γδ T cells are capable of specific recognition, killing of pathogen-infected host cells, regulation of immune responses via lymphokines and initiation of specific antibody production by B cells.

However, most antigens that elicit αß T cell responses fail to stimulate γδ T cells. Furthermore, γδ T cells appear to be distributed mainly in the epithelial layers whereas αß T cells are present in the primary lymphoid organs. To date, it remains unclear whether the responses of γδ T cells are directed specifically against antigen derived from pathogens or from host-derived molecules. However, they are prominent in the acute responses to some bacterial infections, and Mycobacteria are particularly potent inducers of γδ T cell involvement.

II. The Role of Innate Versus Specific Immunity in Infectious Diseases

Depending on the pathogen, non-specific defense components or antigen-specific effectors may play a prominent role. In the case of purulent acute infections (e.g., due to extracellular pathogens), the inflammatory reaction mediated by phagocytes, particularly PMNs and humoral factors, is of major importance.

In contrast, for granulomatous chronic infections caused by facultative or obligate intracellular microorganisms, the host response is classically described as immunologically specific, involving T cells, their products and mononuclear phagocytes, and it corresponds to "cell-mediated" antimicrobial immunity.

This classical picture, however, is exaggeratedly simplified since all components must operate in concert to eradicate infectious agents and to prevent further reinfection.

A. Cooperation Between Innate and Specific Immunity

The cooperation between phagocytes, lymphocytes and humoral factors has been already discussed in the sections on innate and specific immunity (for instance, Ig-dependent phagocytosis). Furthermore, whereas phagocytes possess cytotoxic activities in a non specific manner, a specific pathway has

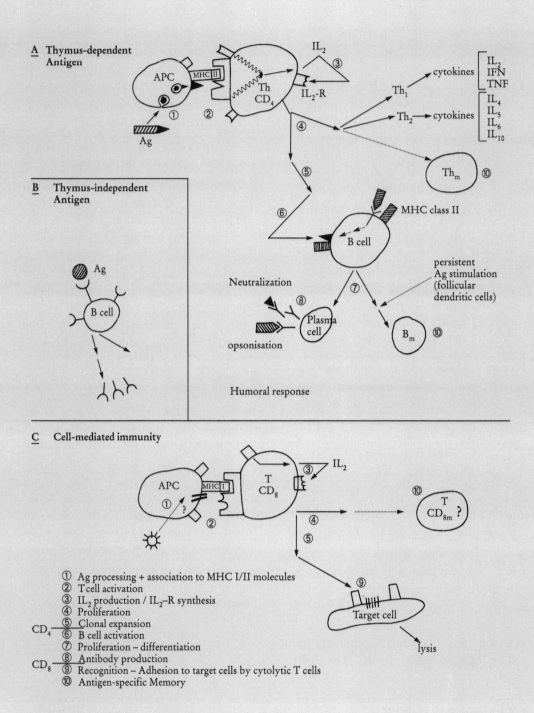

A **Thymus-dependent Antigen**

B **Thymus-independent Antigen**

C **Cell-mediated immunity**

① Ag processing + association to MHC I/II molecules
② T cell activation
③ IL₂ production / IL₂–R synthesis
④ Proliferation
CD₄ ⑤ Clonal expansion
⑥ B cell activation
⑦ Proliferation – differentiation
⑧ Antibody production
CD₈ ⑨ Recognition – Adhesion to target cells by cytolytic T cells
⑩ Antigen-specific Memory

Figure 9 The specific immune response.

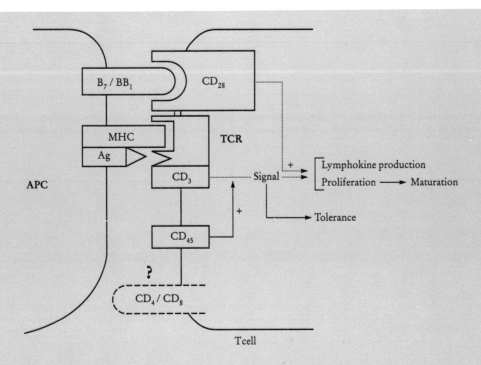

Figure 10 T cell activation during antigen recognition.

been described that directs the cytotoxic activity of phagocytes toward specific targets by means of antibody-dependent cytotoxicity (ADCC) or the killing of specific antibody-opsonized microorganisms.

A major way of coordinating the various effectors in the immune defense is the tremendous panoply of messenger molecules known as the cytokines.

B. Cytokines

The term *cytokines* (CK) covers a wide and still growing number or molecules endowed with cell regulatory properties, also called lymphokines or monokines (depending on their origin), interleukins, interferons and cell-stimulating factors (CSFs). They represent an "intercellular language" and play significant roles in growth, differentiation, host defenses and tissue damages. From the first interleukin (IL-1) discovered in 1972 till the last one, IL-13 (1993), much has been learned about the structure, properties and functions of these factors; the cloning of the CK genes and of most CK receptors, as well as their widespread availability, has led to an explosion of scientific knowledge. CKs, although a heterogeneous group of proteins, have some common characteristics: low molecular weight (<80 kD), glycosylation, transient and local production, effects mediated in a paracrine or autocrine (rather than endocrine) manner, interaction with high-affinity cell surface receptors expressed at a relatively low number (10-10000/cell) and extreme potency (acting at picomolar concentrations). CKs have multiple, overlapping cell regulatory actions. For instance, IL-1, IL-6 and TNF mediate common effects. CKs form a complex network and may induce one another, transmodulate receptors or display synergistic, additive or antagonistic effects on cell functions. This network is under

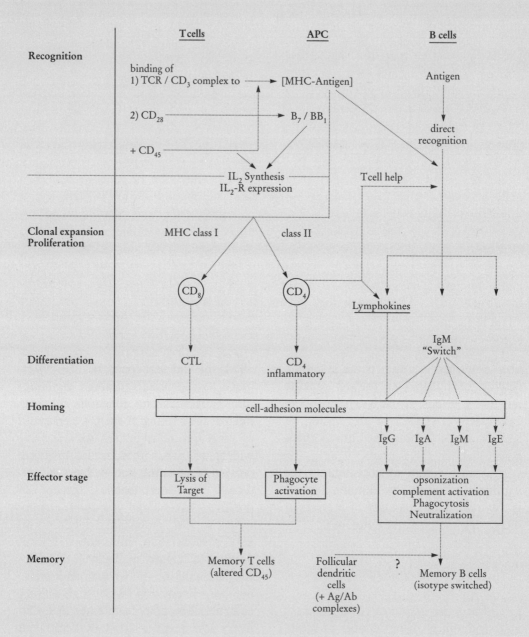

Figure 11 Main steps of the immune response.

complex control at the transcriptional, translational and post translational level. The presence of endogenous CK receptor antagonists (IL-1-Ra, TNF inhibitors, etc.) may provide yet another means of influencing the final response to some CK. At the present time, it is almost impossible to draw a clear picture of CK sequential modulatory pathways in the infectious disease state, since pathogens interfere with various host defense components and different effectors are involved depending on the pathogen.

The various cytokines and their cellular origins, main targets and recognized effects are listed in Table 4. The genes for IL-3, 4, 5, and GM-/M-CSF are located on chromosome 5, those for TNF-α and -β on chromosome 6, IFN-α and -β on chromosome 9, IFN-γ on chromosome 12, IL-1 α and -β on chromosome 2, IL-2 on chromosome 4, IL-6 on chromosome 7, IL-7 on chromosome 8, and G-CSF on chromosome 17.

Whereas cytokines appear to be crucial mediators in host defense to infection, and their potential use in infectious diseases has been suggested by in vivo experimental models, the other side of the coin concerns their deleterious effects when their overproduction may contribute to the pathology of a disease. For instance, TNF seems to play a protective role in experimental murine cutaneous leishmaniasis and activates macrophages and PMNs in vitro to destroy *Leishmania major, Trypanosoma cruzi,* and *Plasmodium falciparum, Entamoeba histolytica,* respectively. On the other hand, TNF has been held responsible for endothelial damage, septic shock and adult respiratory distress syndrome, cerebral malaria and cachexia associated with chronic infections. Similarly, the proinflammatory CK IL-6 is a potent mitogen for mouse plasmocytomas, and recent data provided direct evidence for an autocrine loop in human multiple myeloma.

This double-edged effect of CKs is a general phenomenon of beneficial versus detrimental consequences observed at all levels of natural defense effectors. This has been stressed previously with phagocytes (pathogen destruction versus exaggerated inflammatory response) independently (or not) of CK production, and is also evidenced in lymphocyte biology: T and B cell activation and autoimmune diseases, CTL destruction of infected targets leading to bacterial dissemination (listeriosis) or to tissue damage (Schwann cells and nerve damage in the tuberculoid form of leprosy).

The harmonious coordination of all stages of natural defenses thus appears more critical for optimal anti-infectious efficacy, in which each effector acts in an isolated (even enhanced) manner. Pathogens have developed numerous strategies to survive within their host (see the next chapter), one of which is to dysregulate the harmonious cooperation among all defense components, in particular generating excessive host responses, which in some cases may be the prominent feature of the infectious state.

The possible beneficial/detrimental aspects of host defense effectors are summarized in Table 5.

C. Interregulation Between Specific and Nonspecific Effectors of Host Defenses

Apart for the cytokine network, other molecules may serve as messengers between both the specific and nonspecific immune systems to up/downmodulate cell functions. It has been well demonstrated that phagocytes may regulate their own activity as well as that of lymphocytes and other cells. Some aspects of the various coordinating/regulating pathways between the specific and nonspecific arms of the defense system are illustrated in Figure 12.

Table 4 Cytokines—The State of the Art

Name	Cellular sources	Targets	Effects
IL-1β	Macrophages B, T cells, PMN, epithelial cells, fibroblasts, microglia, keratinocytes, etc.	T, B, stem cells Many other cells	Activation, proliferation, differentiation of T, B, endothelial cells Pyrogenic factor Hepatocyte activating factor Stimulation: osteoclasts, tissue catabolism, production of extracellular matrix protein
IL1-α	Membrane-bound form on macrophages		Antiviral state Proinflammatory (synthesis of PLA2, PGE2, adhesion molecules) Secretion of IL-2, IL-2-R, IL-6 Modulation of hematopoiesis Activation of PMN
IL-2	Activated T cells (TH1)	T, B, cells, LAK, NK, PMN, macrophages	Growth/differentiation cofactor for T, B cells Cytotoxicity NK, LAK
IL-3	Activated TH cells Monocytes Bone marrow stromal cells (?)	Hematopoietic cells	Hematopoietic growth factor (multi-CSF)
IL-4	T cells (TH2)	Hematopoietic cells, T and B cells Thymocytes Macrophages	Growth factor (T, B) Cofactor (+ G-CSF) for erythroid, myeloic, megakaryocytic precursors Increases IgE production Increases HLA class II expression Antagonized by IFN-γ Inhibits IL-2 effects on B cells
IL-5	TH cells (+ IL-2) (TH2)	Hematopoietic cells Eosinophils B cells	Eosinophil differentiation factor Maturation, proliferation of committed B cells into IgA-IgM-producing cells Enhances IL-4 induced IgE synthesis

Table 4 Continued

Name	Cellular sources	Targets	Effects
IL-6	Monocytes Endothelial cells Fibroblasts Some T cell lines (+)	B, T cells Hepatocytes Pluripotent stem cells Plasma cells	Growth factor for GM-CFU (synergy with IL-3) B cell differentiation Growth factor for some transformed B cell lines (EBV, plasmacytoma, hybridoma) Differentiation of myeloid leukemia cell lines Weak antiviral effects Hepatocyte stimulating factor Stimulates T cells (synergy with IL-2, IL-4) Septic shock
IL-7	Stromal bone marrow cells	Pre-B cells Pre-T cells	Growth factor (T, B, thymocytes)
IL-8	Monocytes, PMN (+) → Ala-IL-8 Endothelial cells → Ser-IL-8 Virally infected fibroblasts	PMN (Thy) PMN	Activated PMN (adhesion, migration) Inhibits PMN adhesion
IL-9	T helper cells	Hematopoietic stem cells Erythroid precursors Activated TH Mast cells	Growth factor Stimulates mast cells
IL-10	TH subset (TH2) B cells	B, T cells Macrophages Mast cells	T cell growth factor (ontogeny?) Coinductor cytotoxic T cells Viability B cells, induction of Ia antigens (MHC class II) Inhibits APC function and cytokine synthesis (macrophages) Growth cofactor (mast cells)
IL-11	Bone marrow stromal cell lines	Megakaryocyte precursors	Growth factor (synergy with IL-3)

Table 4 Continued

Name	Cellular sources	Targets	Effects
IL-12	T cells	NK cells, T cells, CTL	Cytotoxic lymphocyte maturation factor Stimulates proliferation of activated T cells Synergy with IL-2→LAK
CLMF (maturation factor for cytotoxic lymphocyte)	B cells	T cells, K, LAK	Enhance T cell proliferation and IFN-γ production Synergy with IL-2 (NK-LAK activation)
TNF-α (cachectin)	LPS-stimulated macrophages T cells (PMN)	Macrophages B cells Endothelial cells Fibroblasts PMN	T, B cell proliferation, differentiation, activation Phagocyte activation Osteoclastic activity Pyrogenic factor Endotoxic shock Necrosis of tumors
TNF-β (lymphotoxin)	T cells (CTL)		Wasting of chronic disease Class I MHC expression Cytolytic activity
TGF	Macrophages	Endothelial cells Fibroblasts Hematopoietic cells B cells	Growth regulation factor (±) synergy with GM-CSF Activate B cells Chemotactic
IFN-α IFN-β IFN-γ	Leukocytes Fibroblasts Activated T cells	Virus-infected cells Tumor cells T cells, macrophages PMN	Antiviral state Inhibit proliferation Activate phagocytes Generate cytotoxic macrophages Activate NK cells Induce class I (IFN-α, -β) or class II (IFN-γ) MHC
S-CSF (kit-ligand soluble membrane-bound)	Bone marrow stromal cells	Hematopoietic precursors	Growth factor

Table 4 Continued

Name	Cellular sources	Targets	Effects
G-CSF	Monocytes, macrophages, fibroblasts, endothelial cells, some leukemic cells lines (bone marrow stromal cells?)	CFU-G PMN, monocytes Some tumor and leukemic cell lines	Myelopoesis Activation of PMN (endothelial cell monocytes)
GM-CSF	T cells, monocytes, fibroblasts, endothelial cells Osteoblasts, some tumor cells (PMN), eosinophils HTLV-I,II-transformed Tly (bone marrow stromal cells?)	Myeloid precursors Erythroid precursors PMN, monocytes, eosinophils, basophils, endothelial cells, tumor, leukemic cell lines	Growth/differentiation factor Activation PMN, macrophages, eosinophils, basophils
M-CSF (3 forms: α, β, γ)	Monocytes (bone marrow stromal cells?)	CFU-M monocytes	Growth and differentiation factor Activation factor
"Small cytokine" superfamily IL-8, NAP-$_2$, MIP2$_\alpha$, MIP2$_\beta$, Gro-MGSA, PF$_4$	Monocytes Various cells Osteoclasts, endothelial cells Fibroblasts	PMN T lymphocytes Hematopoietic cells	Inflammatory properties Modulation hematopoiesis Regulation of immune function Tissue repair, wound healing

Note added in proof: IL-13 is an IL-4-like cytokine that acts on monocytes and B cells, but not on T cells (Zurawski G, De Vries JE, Immunol Today 1994; 15:19–26).

Table 5   **An Attempt to Summarize HDS in Infection**

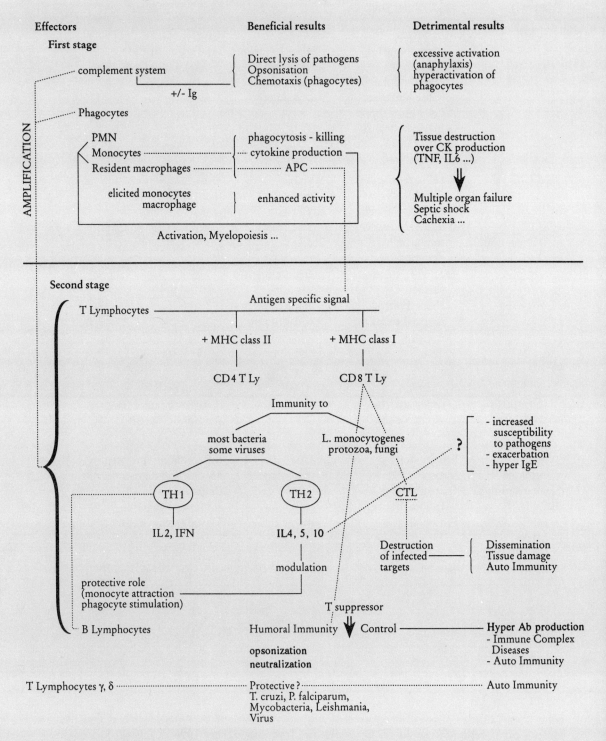

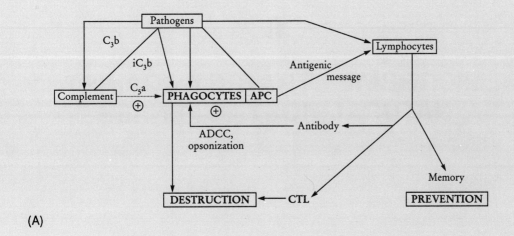

(A)

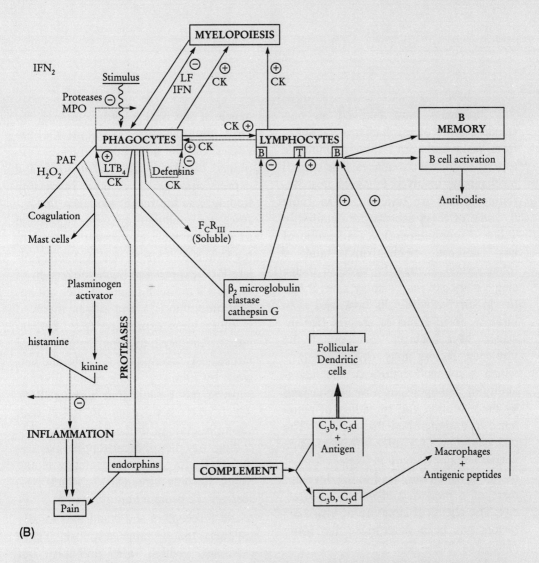

(B)

Figure 12   Some aspects of (A) cooperation and (B) regulation in the immune system.

II

MICROBIAL STRATEGY AGAINST NATURAL HOST DEFENSES

Pathogens have evolved an outstanding array of mechanisms to escape from, resist and even utilize the multiple aspects of immune defenses. The overall mechanisms involved to avoid host defense systems are summarized in Table 6. Some of these aspects are detailed in Tables 7 (complement), 8 (utilization of host defense mechanisms), and 9 (phagocytes). It must be stressed that a single pathogen may display several tactics to survive within its host, and even inside a given genus or species (for instance Mycobacteria, Legionella) the virulence factors may differ strongly, which accounts for the extreme adaptability of pathogens, as now emphasized by the evolution and spreading of resistance to antimicrobial therapeutics. The understanding of virulence mechanisms is now a major domain in bacteriological research, which may lead to the development of a modern anti-infectious strategy. The chemical structure of virulence factors has been determined for some pathogens (Table 10).

Viruses differ from other intracellular pathogens in that their survival within a host cell does not require the mainte-nance of physical integrity. Instead, for virus multiplication to occur, the enzymes of the target cell must be exploited to uncoat the viral genome and express viral genes. A more interesting finding was the recent evidence that viruses can modulate cytokine expression to promote their expression/replication: for instance, TNF-α and IL-6 up-regulate HIV expression. Such subversion of the host's immune response does not appear limited to HIV and may be involved in other virus expression (e.g., herpesvirus). Another intriguing feature is that viruses may manipulate the cytokine network by mimicry: some recent findings concern the Epstein-Barr virus (EBV), which possesses a gene (BCRF-1) with strong homology to the human gene encoding for the immunosuppressive cytokine IL-10. Another example is the Shope fibroma virus (SFV), which possesses a T2 protein homologous to TNF-α and β receptors and could thus locally suppress the immune response. These examples, which are probably not unique, provide an exciting hypothesis to explain virus-induced immunosuppression.

Table 6 Principal Mechanisms of Evasion of Host Defenses by Infectious Agents

Extracorporeal location (toxins)	*Clostridium tetani* *C. botulinum*
Localization in protective niches	Latent syphilis, herpes simplex, latent viral infections (intracellular, genomic situation)
Invasion of cells without lysosomes	*Plasmodium*, *Listeria*, Hemosporidies
Immunosuppression	Most protozoal and viral infections, severe bacterial infections, mycobacteria
Resistance to/inactivation of complement system	Bacteria, protozoa
Inhibition of/escape from phagocyte function	(Intracellular localization, resistance to oxidant stress, bactericidal enzymes, inhibition of chemotaxis, oxidative burst, degranulation)
Utilization of host defenses	Phagocytosis, cytokines
Imitation of host antigens	*Schistosoma*
Antigenic modulation	Malaria, *Leishmania*, *Trypanosoma*
Inappropriate immune response	Lepromatous leprosy, cerebral malaria, endotoxic shock, autoimmunity (Toxoplasma, mycoplasma)

Table 7 Resistance to/Utilization of the Complement System by Pathogens

Pathogens and virulence factors	Consequences
1. Capsules, e.g.	Poor activation of complement Prevent access of phagocytes to C_3b deposited on the cell wall
2. LPS (long side chain)	C_5b-9 generated at distance from the outer membrane

3. *Neisseria*, *T. cruzi* (amastigote),
  Leishmania major
	C_5b-9 does not insert effectively
	  into the lipid bilayer

4. *Streptococcus* sp., *Camphylobacter*,
  Leishmania, Trypanosoma
  (surface structures)
	Interference with C_3 convertase assembly

5. Vaccinia virus (gp 35)
  (homologous to C_4b)
	Mimickry of complement epitope blocks
	  classical pathway C_3 convertase

T. cruzi—gp 160
  (homologous to CR_1, DAF)
	Blocks alternative pathway
	  C_3 convertase

87, 93, 68 kD proteins
  (homologous to CR_1, DAF)
	Blocks assembly/disassembly C_3
	  convertase

? (homologous to C9)	Pore-forming activity (escape into cytoplasm)
C. albicans—165 kD protein (homologous to CR_3)	iC_3b binding)

Table 8 Utilization of Host Defense Mechanisms by Pathogens

I. *Phagocytosis* → **Intracellular localization**

A. *Use of complement receptors*

Pathogen	Infected cells	Receptor
EBV (C_{3dg}-like sequence in gp 350)	B cells	CR_2
Leishmania major gp 63 (RGD sequence)	Monocyte, macrophage	CR_3-CR_4
Leishmania sp.		
deposit of C_3b, iC_3b	Monocyte, macrophage	CR_1-CR_3
lipophosphoglycan	Monocyte, macrophage	CR_3 (lectin-binding site)
L. donovani?	Monocyte, macrophage	CR_3-CR_4
Legionella pneumophila (deposit of C_3b, iC_3b)	Monocyte, macrophage	CR_1-CR_3
Listeria monocytogenes (iC_3b)	Monocyte, macrophage	CR_3
Mycobacterium leprae, *M. tuberculosis* (iC_3b, C_3b)	Monocyte, macrophage	CR_3
C. albicans β glucan, α mannan	Monocyte, macrophage	CR_3 (lectin-binding site)
Histoplasma capsulatum?	Monocyte, macrophage	CR_3, CR_4
HIV C_3b	B, T cells	CR_2
C_3b, iC_3b	Phagocytes	CR_3, CR_4

B. *Use of other receptors to facilitate infection*

M. tuberculosis fibronectin deposit	Phagocyte	FnR
E. coli α-methylmannoside	Phagocyte	FcR_{III}
L. donovani fucose, mannose	Phagocyte	FM-R
H. capsulatum (RGD?)	Phagocyte	LFA_1 (β2 integrin)
HIV gp 120	T cells	CD_4
Antibody deposit (antibody dependent enhancement of viral infectivity)	T, B	FcRII, FcRIII

II. Use of cytokines

Some viruses → inhibition of host response
                → viral replication, expression

Table 9 Microbial Resistance to Phagocytes

1. Toxicity to the phagocytes (leukocidins)	*S. pneumoniae, S. aureus, P. aeruginosa, B. anthracis, E. histolytica*

2. Intracellular localization (facultative/obligate intracellular pathogens)

Phagosome (inhibition of degranulation)	Cytoplasm (escape into)	Phagolysosome (resistance to killing systems)
N. asteroides	Viruses	*Y. pestis*
M. tuberculosis, M. microti, M. avium	*M. leprae* *T. cruzi*	*H. capsulatum* *C. burnetii*
C. psittaci, C. trachomatis	Rickettsiae	*Leishmania major*
T. gondii	*L. monocytogenes*	*L. donovani*
B. abortus (depending on virulence)	*S. flexneri*	*M. lepraemurium*
L. pneumophila (strain Philadelphia)		*L. pneumophila* *L. micdadei*
Leishmania brasiliensis		*A. fumigatus*
Chlorella sp.		*S. typhimurium*

3. Inhibition of phagocyte function

Chemotaxis	Adherence ingestion	Oxidative burst
S. typhi	Pasteurella, Mycoplasma	*S. typhi*
N. meningitidis	Neisseria	*B. abortus*
N. gonorrheae		Borrelia
E. coli	*E. coli*	Leishmania
S. aureus	*S. aureus*	
Serratia	*Y. pestis*	*T. gondii*
M. tuberculosis	*S. pneumoniae*	*T. cruzi*
	B. fragilis	

4. Resistance to killing systems

Oxidative stress	Oxygen-independent systems
E. coli, S. aureus, L. monocytogenes, B. abortus, N. asteroides, Leishmania, M. leprae, S. lutea	*S. typhimurium* *S. minnesota* *M. leprae*

Table 10 Examples of Virulence Factors

Pathogen	Structure	Effect
Mycobacteria sp.	Lipoarabinomannan	Interference with priming/activation of phagocytes
M. leprae	Phenolic glycolipid	Scavenges oxygen metabolites
Leishmania sp.	Lipophosphoglycan	Scavenges oxygen metabolites, inhibits protein kinase C
Listeria monocytogenes	Listeriolysin 58 kD	Transition from endosomal to cytoplasmic compartment
	Protein 60 kD	Entry into phagocytes
Rickettsia	Phospholipase A	Escape into cytoplasm

III

IMMUNODEFICIENCIES

Progress in therapeutics, medicine and surgery had revealed — and sometimes created — a new category of patients who are "immunocompromised" and at a high risk for developing infectious diseases. These immunodeficiencies may be congenital, involving one or more effectors of the natural defenses, or acquired secondary to various pathological states and associated therapeutics. This immunodeficient state favors infection by opportunistic pathogens (which are often resistant to classic antibacterial agents), as well as difficult-to-treat polymicrobial infections. Even appropriate antimicrobial therapy proves unsuccessful in a large number of these patients, who thus represent a therapeutic challenge for the next century. Our under-standing of the pathogenesis of immunodeficiency diseases at the cellular and molecular levels is progressing, and this should permit us to modulate specific components of the immune system by the use of biologic response modifiers.

The various immunodeficiencies are summarized in Tables 11–19 and their infectious consequences in Tables 20 and 21.

It must be underlined that many acquired immunodeficiencies involve more than one specific effector and that immune status can evolve during the course of infections with sequential phagocyte activation/deactivation events, complement consumption and inflammatory cytokine production.

Table 11   Classification of Immune Deficiency Disorders

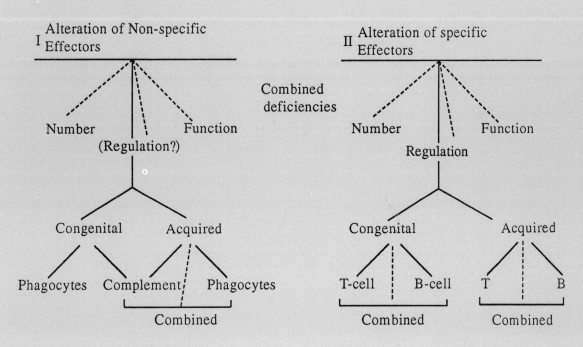

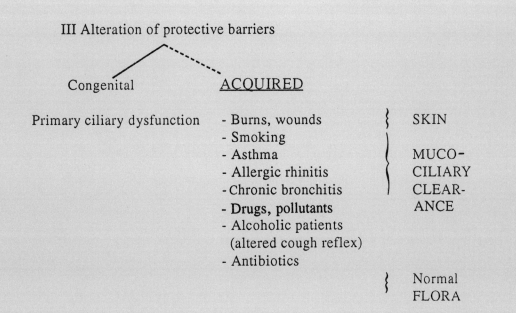

Table 12 Primary Complement Deficiencies

Defective component	Frequency	Consequences
C19	≥40 cases	Pyogenic infections
C1r, C1s	10	Meningitis
C4	17	Systemic lupus erythematosus
C2	≥100	Many healthy people
C3	16	Glomerulonephritis
Alternative pathway activation systems	1–≥50	Neisserial infections (rare pyogenic infection)
Terminal components C5-9	19–≥50	Neisserial infections

Table 13 Neutropenia (NE) Classification

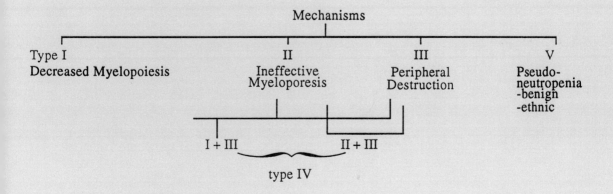

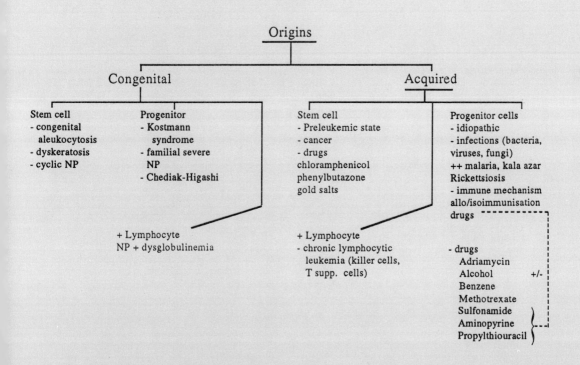

Table 14   Drugs and Neutropenia (for effects of antibiotics, see Table 24)

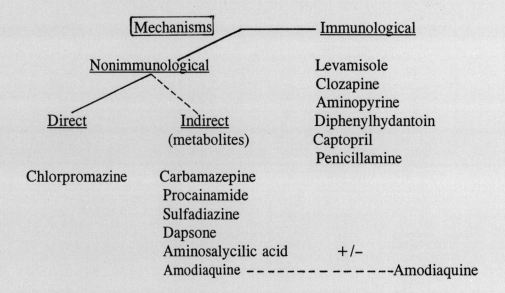

Table 15 Phagocyte Dysfunction

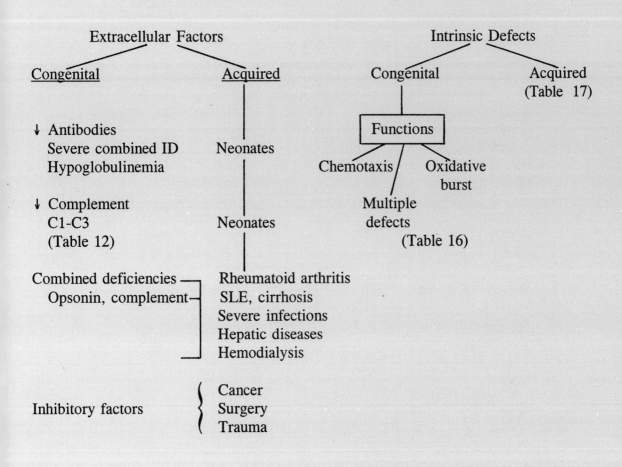

Table 16 Congenital Defects of PMN Functions

Chemotaxis	Oxidative burst	Combined defects
Chediak-Higashi	Chronic granulomatous	Leukocyte adhesion
Kartagener syndrome	disease (CGD) $1/10^6$	deficiency (adhesion,
Juvenile periodontitis	births, defect of the	chemotaxis,
	NADPH oxidase system	phagocytosis, ~60 cases)
	Autosomal recessive ~35%	Specific granule
	X-linked ~66%	deficiency (chemotaxis,
		killing) defensins ↓
	MPO deficiency	
	1/2000 births	
	G$_6$PD deficiency	
	Gluthathion peroxidase	
	Gluthathion synthetase	
	Glycogenosis 1b	

Table 17   Acquired PMN Dysfunctions

		Extrinsic factors
I.	Systemic diseases	
	Diabetes mellitus	Ketoacidosis
	↓ adhesion, phagocytosis	Hyperosmolarity
	→ infections (fungal, pyogenic)	Urinary glucose?
	Renal impairment	↓ C5a, opsonins
	CAPD, hemodialysis	
	→ peritonitis (S. epidermidis)	
	Cirrhosis, uremia	Anemia
		Altered hepatic function
		(synthesis of
		complement)
		Hypersplenism
	Monoclonal immunoglobulin	Decreased antibodies
II.	Myeloproliferative diseases	Inhibitory factors
	± granulopenia	
III.	Drugs	
	Steroids, NSAIDS	
	Anticancer chemotherapy	
	Antibiotics (in vitro)	
IV.	Surgery, trauma, burns,	↓ Opsonins, complement
	cyclic decrease of PMN bactericidal functions	inhibitors
	Deactivated PMN-degranulation (release	Parenteral nutrition
	of MPO) → infection	↓ T/B lymphocytes
	"Priming" → ARDS, septic shock	
V.	Bacterial, viral, protozoal infection	T/B dysfunction
	± neutropenia	
	↗ priming → septic shock	
	↘ deactivation → superinfections	
VI.	Chronic bronchitis, psoriasis, Crohn's disease	
	activation, degranulation → tissue damage	
VII.	Age: Neonates–premature: ↓ PMN adherence,	
	bactericidal function, autooxidative damage	Decreased Ig
	Malnutrition stress (++depression)	Decreased opsonins

Table 18   Primary Immunodeficiencies

1) Mechanisms

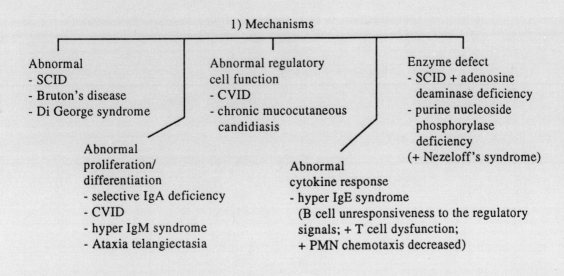

Abnormal
- SCID
- Bruton's disease
- Di George syndrome

Abnormal regulatory
cell function
- CVID
- chronic mucocutaneous
  candidiasis

Enzyme defect
- SCID + adenosine
  deaminase deficiency
- purine nucleoside
  phosphorylase
  deficiency
  (+ Nezeloff's syndrome)

Abnormal
proliferation/
differentiation
- selective IgA deficiency
- CVID
- hyper IgM syndrome
- Ataxia telangiectasia

Abnormal
cytokine response
- hyper IgE syndrome
  (B cell unresponsiveness to the regulatory
  signals; + T cell dysfunction;
  + PMN chemotaxis decreased)

2) Targets

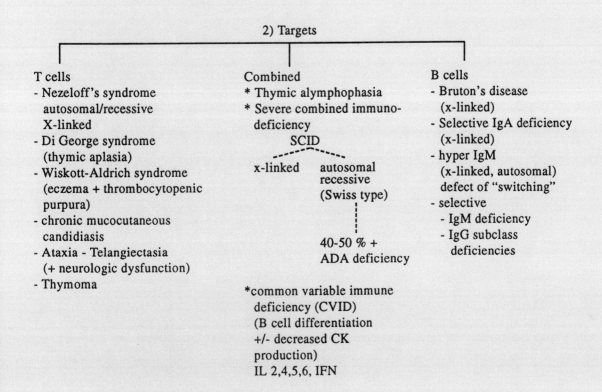

T cells
- Nezeloff's syndrome
  autosomal/recessive
  X-linked
- Di George syndrome
  (thymic aplasia)
- Wiskott-Aldrich syndrome
  (eczema + thrombocytopenic
  purpura)
- chronic mucocutaneous
  candidiasis
- Ataxia - Telangiectasia
  (+ neurologic dysfunction)
- Thymoma

Combined
* Thymic alymphophasia
* Severe combined immuno-
  deficiency

    SCID

x-linked   autosomal
           recessive
           (Swiss type)

        40-50 % +
        ADA deficiency

*common variable immune
 deficiency (CVID)
 (B cell differentiation
 +/- decreased CK
 production)
 IL 2,4,5,6, IFN

B cells
- Bruton's disease
  (x-linked)
- Selective IgA deficiency
  (x-linked)
- hyper IgM
  (x-linked, autosomal)
  defect of "switching"
- selective
  - IgM deficiency
  - IgG subclass
    deficiencies

Table 19   Acquired Specific Immunodeficiency

Age: Neonates: ↓ B-cell differentiation, Ig production
     Old people: impaired T-cell function→ infections, cancer, autoimmunity
                   (GVH, DTH, MLR)

Hematologic lymphoproliferative disorders⎫
   Hodgkin's disease—lymphoma   ⎬ Infiltration of bone marrow
   Leukemia
   Myeloma, macroglobulinemia   (+ therapeutics)
   Agranulocytosis—Aplastic anaemia
   Sickle cell disease   ↓ Antibody production

Systemic disease
   Nephrotic syndrome   ↓ Ig levels
   Protein-losing enteropathy
   Malnutrition   Impairment of cellular immunity

Surgery, trauma, burns, splenectomy   T-cell subsets changes

Immunosuppressive agents
   Antimetabolites
   Corticosteroids
   Radiation

Pregnancy   T-cell subsets changes
   Hormones? proteins?
   Increased susceptibility to viruses,
     protozoa

Cancer
   Therapeutics
   Circulating inhibitors
   Infiltration of bone marrow   Impairment of cell-mediated immunity
   Surgery
   Parenteral nutrition

Viral infections
   AIDS opportunistic infections   ↓ ThCD4 (+ ↓ macrophage function)

Table 20 Infectious Consequences of Primary Immunodeficiencies

Defect	Onset of infection	Infection characteristics
S.C.I.D.	First 6 months of life	Overwhelming, life-threatening bacterial, viral, fungal infections → fatal outcome
Bruton's disease	First 2 years	Recurrent sinopulmonary infections (pneumococci, streptococci, Haemophilus)
Nezeloff syndrome	Early	Recurrent skin, urinary, pulmonary infections, cutaneous candidiasis, severe progressive varicella
Di George syndrome	Early	Severe to mild infections
Selective IgA deficiency		Few infections (respiratory tract) (+ allergy, asthma, autoimmunity)
CVI	Adults	Recurrent sinopulmonary infections
Hyper IgM		Recurrent pyogenic infections (+ autoimmunity)
Ataxia-telangiectasia	Early	Recurrent sinopulmonary infections
Wiskott-Aldrich syndrome	Early (1st year)	Otitis media, pneumonia, meningitis ± sepsis (+++ encapsulated pathogen)
	Later	*P. carinii*, herpesvirus, e.g. → fatal (malignancy 12%)
Chronic mucocutaneous candidiasis		*Candida albicans* (± bacteria) infections
Hyper IgE syndrome		Infections with *S. aureus* (++), *H. influenzae*, pneumococci, gram-negative organisms, *C. albicans*
Purine nucleoside phosphorylase deficiency	Early	Opportunistic infections, generalized vaccinia, varicella (+ lymphosarcoma)
Complement deficiency		e.g.; Neisseria infections (see Table 12)
Neutropenia		e.g.; Multiple severe infections, fatal prognosis, except congenital dyskeratosis: mild infection; cyclic NP: moderate to severe infections
PMN dysfunctions		
CGD	Early	Severe pyogenic, fungal infections (+ granuloma formation)
MPO deficiency	Late	Rare infections; some *C. albicans* (+ cancer)
LAD	Early	Severe to mild infections (pyogenic, fungal + impaired wound healing)

Table 21 Specific/Non-specific Immune Dysfunctions and
Infections

Origin	Pathogens
Phagocyte Neutropenia Dysfunction	Bacteria: *S. aureus*, *S. epidermidis*, *E. coli*, *K. pneumoniae*, Enterobacteriaceae, *P. aeruginosa* Fungi: Candida sp., Aspergillus, Mucor sp. Virus: Herpes simplex
Complement	Neisseria
Cellular immunity	Bacteria: Listeria, Salmonella sp., Mycobacteria, Legionella, *Nocardia asteroides* Fungi: *Cryptococcus neoformans*, Candida sp., Histoplasma, *Coccidioides immitis* Virus: Herpes, varicella-zoster, cytomegalovirus, hepatitis A, B Protozoa: *P. carinii*, *T. gondii*, *Giardia lamblia*, *E. histolytica*, Cryptosporidium enteritis Worms: *Strongyloides stercoralis*
Humoral immunity	Bacteria: *Streptococus pneumoniae*, *Haemophilus influenzae*

IV

FUNCTIONAL AND CHRONOBIOLOGICAL VARIATIONS OF IMMUNE DEFENSE

A final point is that most relevant data have established a static picture, which is far from what occurs in the host. It is now clear that:

1. There is an extreme interindividual variability in the functional capacity of natural defenses.

2. Functional responses vary according to external factors and cyclic chronobiological changes.

Interindividual variability of phagocyte number, functions and sensitivity to drugs has been evidenced in many studies. Similarly, the broad range of immunoglobulin and complement levels, the percentage and functional activity of T cell subsets also suggests variation at the specific immune response level. The basis of such variability is unknown. Although, sex, age, and race-related differences exist, other phenomena under genomic control are likely. This could explain the particular sensitivity of some individuals to infections, as observation also made in genetically controlled animal models.

The intraindividual variability of host defenses is also widely recognized. For instance, PMNs are often studied as a single-cell population but not only can their functions differ according to the cell pool analyzed (bone marrow reserve granulocytes, circulating or marginated granulocyte pools) but functional differences are found between the various subsets, of the same pool, although this has not been as well analyzed as T cells. Furthermore, environmental factors such as physical and psychological stress, seasonal influences and circadian rhythms may modify their tissue distribution and functional activity. The chronobiology of specific im-

Table 22 The "Immune Clock"

	Optimal timing
NK cell activity	8 and 20 h
CD3, CD4 lymphocyte	8 h
T-cell activation (PHA)	6–10 h
Latent activation	12–18 h
Cell proliferation	
Bone marrow (DNA synthesis)	16–20 h
Peripheral blood lymphocytes	8–10 h and 20–24 h
Lymphocyte release into blood	
B-cells	20–24 h
T-cells	24–4 h

mune functions is becoming a major research area, although most data are being obtained in animal models. Some studies do, however, refer to circadian rhythms in human T and B proliferation, NK activity and phagocytic functions; immune defenses also seem to be organized along other time scales: a depression of T cell immunity occurs in winter but does not appear to be related to light or temperature (in animal models). Other periodicities — circamenstrual (about 30 days) and circaseptan (about 7 days) — also modulate the immune response, as shown in premenopausal women with breast cancer and transplant patients, respectively. Some aspects of the immune clock in humans are shown in Table 22.

These immunological rhythms are of major importance to optimize therapeutics, in particular when biological response modifiers are considered. Chronotherapy is already used in the treatment of cancer to minimize toxic side effects of drugs, and some phase I clinical trials with immunomodulators (IFN-α) suggest that time-adaptable drug delivery would improve their therapeutic index. Circadian studies of the efficacy of anti-infectious agents may be a significant future trend in antimicrobial research.

V

NEW TRENDS IN THE TREATMENT OF INFECTIOUS DISEASES

With the spread of resistance to the most modern anti-infective drugs, new strategies are obviously required. They include improvements in pharmacokinetics, bacterial spectrum and potency, as well as decreased toxic side effects and the search for new antibacterial mechanisms, new classes of anti-infective drugs (magainins, antisense oligonucleotides) or new vehicles (liposomes; "antibiobodies," i.e., antimicrobial immunoglobulins). Also of major importance is the restoration of compromised natural effectors. Gene therapy may prove effective, but this is highly selective and reserved for very few patients. Various combinations of antimicrobials and immunomodulators are already undergoing clinical trials. The efficacy of CSFs (G-CSF, GM-CSF) to restore granulocyte numbers after anticancer chemotherapy or bone marrow engraftment, and in genetic or acquired granulocytopenic states, is clear. Their use in infections still needs further studies.

A seducing therapeutic approach to infectious states concerns the development of antimicrobial molecules endowed with immunomodulatory properties. This is analyzed in the following chapter.

Anti-Infective Agents and the Immune System

As soon as anti-infective drugs entered the therapeutic armamentarium, their possible interference with the host natural defenses was suggested. In the late 19th century, Metchnikoff and Helmholz and their respective co-workers analyzed the effects of quinine, and found that it enhanced phagocytosis (Metchnikoff) and decreased inflammatory reactions (Helmholz). This dual aspect of a given molecule depending on the dose and experimental conditions is one factor that renders so complex the analysis of a possible modulation of host defenses by antibiotics.

To date, a large amount of data are available concerning the possible "immunomodulatory" properties of most antibacterial agents, and despite intense controversies, related to laboratory conditions, some general conclusions may be drawn. The main points of interaction between antibacterial agents and the host defense system are schematized in Figure 13, and the desired characteristics of a suitable antibacterial agent with immunomodulating properties are listed in Table 23.

First, antibacterial agents may alter the number of immunocompetent cells at the level of generation, proliferation and differentiation of the lympho- and monomyelocytic lineage. Published data refer mainly to depressive effects with secondary consequences in vivo, in particular agranulocytosis (Table 24). Other immunorelated side effects concern allergic reactions associated with the use of some antibacterial agents (Table 25).

Second, they may alter directly of indirectly the host defense system. Previous alterations of microorganisms and their virulence factors may result in indirect modifications of natural defenses, e.g., increased stimulatory activity of the altered pathogens for phagocytes and/or increased susceptibility to bactericidal systems, decreased production of various virulence factors (toxins, capsule, other antiphagocytic structures, protein M, protein A, etc.) and even modification of immunogenicity (Table 26). These indirect effects of antibacterial agents are demonstrated for most molecules in vitro, but experimental models of infection suggest that they could also be effective in vivo.

A direct modification of host natural defenses by antibacterial agents is more speculative. Although some drugs may alter phagocyte or lymphocyte function in vitro (and, for some of these anti-infective drugs, the mechanisms of inhibition/enhancement have been elucidated), the data obtained ex vivo are less numerous and the relevance to the clinical situation is still uncertain. Some of the problems in interpreting in vitro, ex

vivo and in vivo results are summarized in Table 27, and the results themselves are given in Table 28.

A clinically relevant and now widely admitted effect of anti-infective drugs on the host defense system is the property of some of them to concentrate actively inside phagocytes and to display intracellular bioactivity that permits eradication of facultative/obligate intracellular pathogens (Table 29). Apart from this direct antibacterial efficacy, a possible consequence of drug entry into phagocytes is the synergy that may occur between the antibacterial agent and the natural bactericidal systems (enzymes and oxidant stress). This synergy may be related either to a drug-induced modification of the susceptibility of microorganisms to phagocyte killing (or conversely to a phagocyte-induced increased sensitivity of microorganisms to the drugs) or to a modification of the drug leading to altered and more potent bactericidal molecules, or to a synergy between natural and therapeutic bactericidal systems (Table 28).

Finally, drugs can be modified by phagocytes themselves or by metabolic pathways and generate toxic molecules leading to tissue damage and host cell destruction.

When all these points are considered, a somewhat simplified picture may be drawn (Figure 14) to classify anti-infective drugs according to their effects on the host defense system. It thus appears clearly that the cupboard of "antimicrobial-immune response modifier [IRM] agents" is rather bare.

Recently, a molecule belonging to the "third-generation" cephalosporins, cefodizime, has been reported to be a good candidate. Why this aminothiazolyl is considered the forerunner of a new class of antibacterial drugs is the subject of the last chapter in this review.

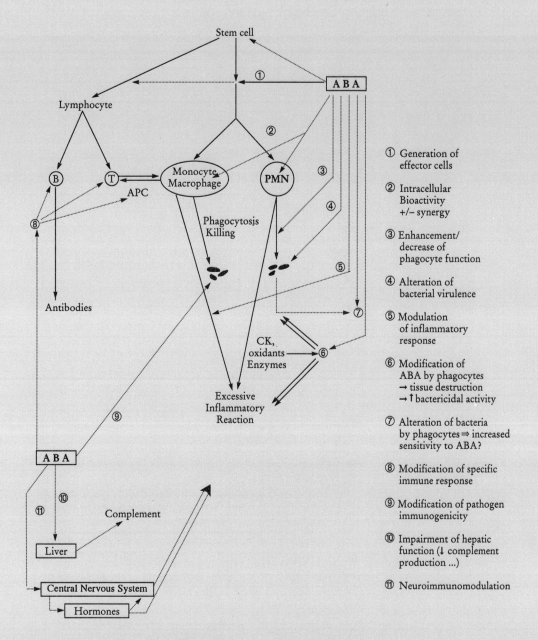

Stem cell

ABA

Lymphocyte

① Generation of
effector cells

B T
APC

Monocyte
Macrophage

PMN

② Intracellular
Bioactivity
+/− synergy

③ Enhancement/
decrease of
phagocyte function

Phagocytosis
Killing

④ Alteration of
bacterial virulence

⑤ Modulation
of inflammatory
response

Antibodies

CK,
oxidants
Enzymes

⑥ Modification of
ABA by phagocytes
→ tissue destruction
→ ↑ bactericidal activity

Excessive
Inflammatory
Reaction

⑦ Alteration of bacteria
by phagocytes ⇒ increased
sensitivity to ABA?

⑧ Modification of specific
immune response

⑨ Modification of pathogen
immunogenicity

ABA

Complement

⑩ Impairment of hepatic
function (↓ complement
production ...)

⑪ Neuroimmunomodulation

Liver

Central Nervous System

Hormones

Figure 13 Antibacterial agents and the immune system.

Table 23 Desired Characteristics of Immunomodulatory Antibacterial Agents
(*antibacterial effect)

1. No immunologic side effects: allergy, myelopoiesis
2. Haematopoiesis: enchanced proliferation - generation of monomyelocytic lineage

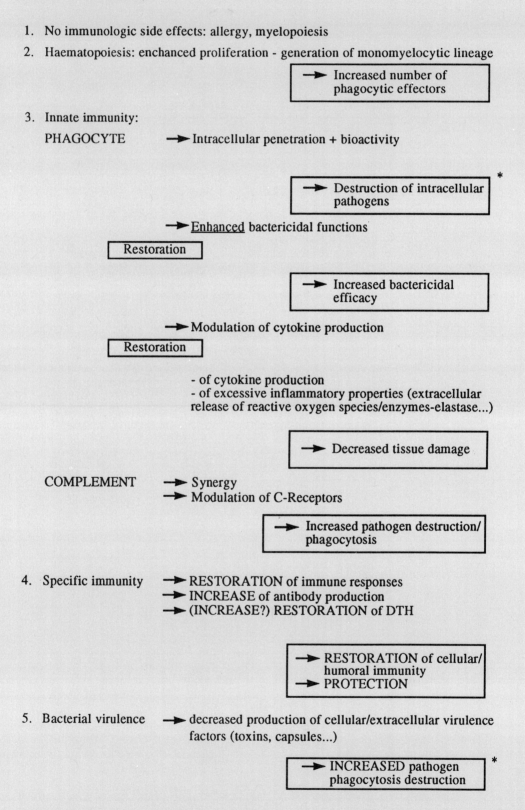

3. Innate immunity:
   PHAGOCYTE → Intracellular penetration + bioactivity

   → Destruction of intracellular pathogens *

   → Enhanced bactericidal functions
   Restoration

   → Increased bactericidal efficacy

   → Modulation of cytokine production
   Restoration

   - of cytokine production
   - of excessive inflammatory properties (extracellular
   release of reactive oxygen species/enzymes-elastase...)

   → Decreased tissue damage

   COMPLEMENT → Synergy
   → Modulation of C-Receptors

   → Increased pathogen destruction/ phagocytosis

4. Specific immunity → RESTORATION of immune responses
   → INCREASE of antibody production
   → (INCREASE?) RESTORATION of DTH

   → RESTORATION of cellular/ humoral immunity
   → PROTECTION

5. Bacterial virulence → decreased production of cellular/extracellular virulence
   factors (toxins, capsules...)

   → INCREASED pathogen phagocytosis destruction *

Table 24 Antibiotics That May Induce Neutropenia

Methicillin, oxacillin, ampicillin, carbenicillin
Chloramphenicol
Gentamicin
Isoniazid
Rifampicin
Sulfonamides
Ciprofloxacin (+TNF)

Table 25 Allergic Reactions to Anti-Infective Drugs

Mechanisms	Drugs	
IgE-mediated hypersensitivity (anaphylaxis)	Frequent:	Penicillin G—other β-lactams (cross-reaction) Clindamycin, dapsone, gentamicin, isoniazid, streptomycin, nitrofurantoin, sulfonamides, trimethoprim-sulfamethoxazole
	Occasional:	Amikacin, chloramphenicol, ethambutol, ethionamide, ketoconazole, lincomycin, nalidixic acid, rifampicin, trimethoprim
Cytotoxic antibodies		
Immune hemolytic anemia	Penicillin, cephalosporin, quinine, quinidine	
Thrombocytopenia	Quinine, quinidine, sulfonamides	
Granulocytopenia	Sulfonamides, antimalarial drugs	
Antigen-Antibody complexes (serum thickness)	Penicillin, sulfonamides, streptomycin	
Cell-mediated hypersensitivity		
Contact dermatitis	Neomycin	
Lung	Nitrofurantoin, penicillin	
Presumed immunologic drug reaction		
Skin eruption, Stevens-Johnson syndrome, Lyell's syndrome	Penicillin, sulfonamides	
Hepatic hypersensitivity	Sulfonamides, isoniazid, erythromycin estolate	
Renal hypersensitivity	Penicillin G, methicillin	

Skin test reactions (frequency)			
Amoxicillin	5.14%	INH	0.56%
TMP-SMX	3.38%	Doxycycline	0.47%
Ampicillin	3.32%	Gentamycin sulfate	4.5%
Cephalosporin	2.11%		
Erythromycin	2.04%		
Penicillin G	1.95%		

Source: Anderson S. A. et al., JAMA 1987; 258:2891.

Table 26 Indirect Effects of Antibacterial Agents on the Host Defense System
(e.g., assessed in vitro)

Effects	Antibacterial Agents	Bacteria
Enhanced susceptibility to oxidative stress/enzymes of phagocytes (± complement)	Most β-lactams[a]	Sensitive strains
	Some β-lactams	Resistant strains
	Clindamycin/lincomycin	Senstitive/Resistant strains
	Polymyxin B, colistin	
	Aminoglycoside	
	Chloramphenicol	Enterobacteriaceae
	Tetracyclin	
	Macrolides	
	Sulfisoxazole	Sensitive strains
	Vancomycin	
Enhanced stimulation	Most β-lactams	Sensitive/Resistant strains
	Macrolides	*H. influenzae, S. aureus*
	Quinolones	*S. aureus*
Altered virulence factors	Erythromycin	*P. aeruginosa* (leucotoxin)
	Clindamycin	Protein A (*S. aureus*)
		Protein M (*S. pyogenes*)
	Macrolides	Adherence factors
	Quinolones	(sensitive strains)
Immune reactivity	Quinolones	↓ Immunogenicity *E. coli*
LPS release	Quinolones	*E. coli*

[a] Demonstrated also in vivo (experimental models of infections).

Table 27 Analysis of Interactions Between Antibacterial Agents and the Host Defense System: Methodologic Problems

In vitro	Ex vivo	In vivo
Technique		Only model available =
Dose/nature of stimulus		experimental
Animal species		infections
Nature/state of the cells		1) Animals≠humans
PMN-monocyte-macrophage primed-elicited-resting?	Idem	2) Animals
Lymphocyte subsets ...		Strain A≠strain B
Interindividual sensitivity		Pharmacokinetics
Chronobiology		Metabolism
Environmental factors		Chronobiology
Healthy/Immunocompromised animals/humans		Immune system ...
Drug concentration	Drug dose/ Administration route/time	
Artefacts oxidant scavenging/ production by the drug?	Removal of drug/ immune byproducts	

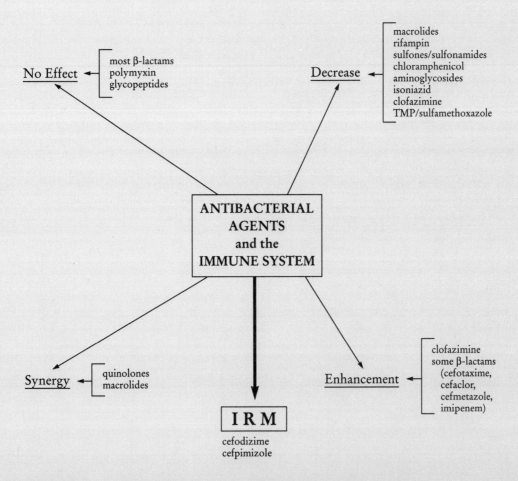

Figure 14 Antibacterial agents and the host defense system.

Table 28 Direct Effects of Antibacterial Agents on the Host Defense System In Vitro (therapeutic concentrations)

Increase	Decrease
Cefmetazole ⎫	
Cefpimizole ⎬ phagocyte functions	
Cefodizime ⎭	Cephalothin (IL-2)
Cefotaxime (PMN)	Cefotaxime (macrophages)
Macrolides	Josamycin (Ab production)
Roxithromycin ⎫ phagocytosis	Some macrolides (oxidant production)
Josamycin ⎬ bacterial killing	Amphotericin B (PMN)
Spiramycin (IL-6 production)	Ciprofloxacin (CSF production,
Amphotericin B (macrophages)	synergy with TNF-IFN-γ)
Clindamycin (PMN killing—low dose)	Rifampicin (+ artefacts)
Ciprofloxacin (IFN-γ production)	PMN chemotaxis,
	oxygen radical formation
	Lymphocyte responsiveness
	to mitogens
	Cyclins (PMN functions,
	mitogen responsiveness)
	Antimalarial drugs (PMN)
	Isoniazid
	Pentamidine salts
	Fusidic acid
	Sulfonamides

Ex vivo

Cefodizime (various functions)	Josamycin
Cefpimizole (PMN functions)	(PMN chemotaxis, Ab production)
Cefaclor (MPO activity)	Tetracyclins
Erythromycin (PMN chemotaxis)	
Roxithromycin (PMN functions)	

In vivo →
(experimental models of infection)

Cefodizime	Cefoxitin

→ Idiosyncratic reaction–toxicity
(see Tables 24 and 25)

Table 29 Intracellular Bioactivity of Anti-Infectious Agents

Drugs	Cellular/Extracellular Ratio		Bioactivity (intracellular bacteria)	Localization
	PMN	Macrophages		
β-Lactams	e.g. ≪1		+? Penicillin G	Membrane-associated?
Aminoglycosides	≤1		+? Depends on the bacteria	Membrane slow (2-3 days) intracellular penetration → granule
Quinolones	2–8	2–8	+	Primarily cytoplasmic
Macrolides	15–79	17–120 (↑ in smokers)	± Depends on the strain and the macrolide	PMN granules 13–33 % + cytoplasm
Clindamycin	10–40	23–50	(+)	Granules?
Rifampicin	2–8	5–10	+	
Rifapentin	88	62	+	
Chloramphenicol	3–10	2	+?	Membrane?
Lincomycin	1–6	2	(+)?	
INH	1–3		?	
Trimethoprim	6–13		(+)	
Teicoglanin	52	41	?	
Tetracycline	0.75	2.4		Nucleus
Polymyxin B	Hela cells		(+)?	
Sulfonamides	1.7–3.4			

VI

CEFODIZIME TODAY AND TOMORROW: RESULTS AND PROMISES

As emphasized previously, many hopes for anti-infective strategy are now based on the potential use of two-edged therapeutic swords (anti-infective + IRM), offering the advantage of single administration, the same pharmacokinetics, and tissue distribution (as long as both activities occur at similar concentrations!).

Some antibiotics may favor one or more antibacterial defense systems (e.g., phagocytosis). However, to be included in the IRM category, molecules should have a clear impact on the whole host defense system, manifested at various specific/nonspecific immune levels. Cefodizime had been the subject of extensive reviews, and at the present time it appears to be the only molecule that alters the specific/nonspecific immune system in multiple ways. Furthermore, the chemical structure responsible for such IRM activity has been identified as the thiothiazolyl moiety attached at position 3 of the cephem ring (Figure 15). The structure has been modified and the resulting molecule (HBW 538—Tiproti-

mod) can provoke immunological responses; it should be a promising drug in fields other than infectious diseases. The data concerning the immunomodulatory effects of cefodizime are summarized in Tables 30–33.

Many points need further evaluation to better assess the IRM activity of cefodizime in infectious diseases:

1. The precise mechanism underlying the observed effects is not yet understood. The possible stimulating effect on the release of "cytokine" (?) or other factor(s) has not been fully explored and the "mediator(s)" involved (if any) are yet undefined.

2. The chronobiology-dependent activity of cefodizime shown in some models has not been taken into account in most experimental studies, and this may explain some controversial results. As stressed previously, this research area is be-

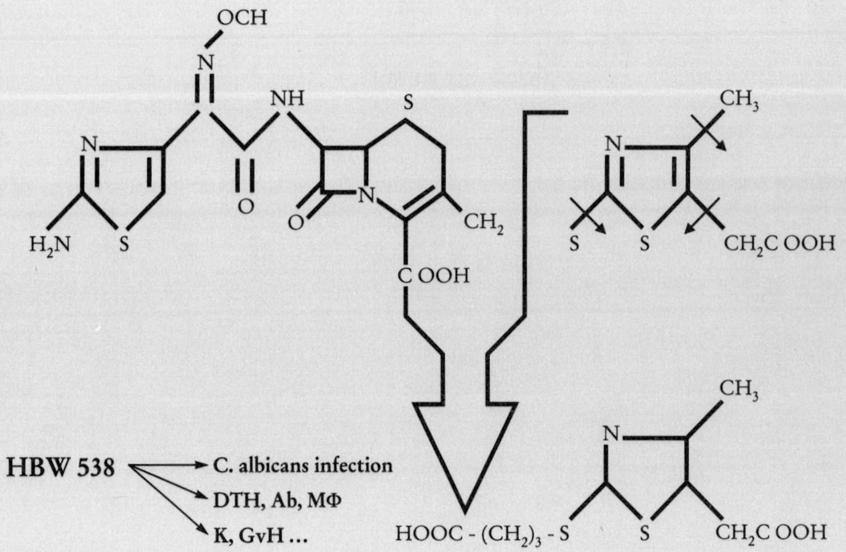

Figure 15 Immune "enhancer" chemical structure of cefodizime.

coming essential in the full exploitation of immune modulators.

3. The strain-species dependence of IRM activity in some experiments (infection models, lymphocyte function etc.) is also a crucial point in the design of future studies. This is true not only of cefodizime but also of amphotericin B in macrophages of high/low-responder mouse strains. The problem is of major importance when comparing the effect of any drug on the defense system of humans and animals (see Table 27).

Taken as a whole, the data presented here show that cefodizime deeply alters various immunological parameters in vitro, ex vivo and in vivo. The most constant finding is the potentiation of phagocyte response, in particular phagocytosis and bactericidal activity. It also restores in vitro and ex vivo some phagocyte functions such as chemotaxis and the oxidative burst. More interesting is the fact that cefodizime up/down-modulates cytokine production ex vivo (restoration of IL-1 and TFN production in immunocompromised animals) and in vitro (inhibition of IL-1 and TNF release by LPS-stimulated monocytes).

The cefodizime interaction with the specific immune response system has been found mainly ex vivo in experimental models and depends on the animal species/strain, duration of treatment, etc. This strongly favours the hypothesis that the primary action of cefodizime involves phagocytes (possibly through specific membrane binding) and results in the release of one or more mediators acting on lymphocyte functions.

Cefodizime interference with the host defense system during the course of infectious diseases is schematized in Figure 16.

Acknowledgment

The author wishes to thank Miss Fr. Breton for expert secretarial assistance.

Table 30   In Vivo IRM Activity of Cefodizime (experimental models of infection)

Model	Microorganism	Results
A) Resistant pathogens		
1. Prophylactic administration		
<u>Septicemia</u>		
Balb/c mice $\Big\{$	*C. albicans*	Enhanced survival
	T. gondii	Comparators $\Big\{$ latamoxef (no effect) cefoperazone
Swiss mice →	*P. berghei* →	Enhanced survival (Circadian-dependent effect)
NMRI mice →	*C. albicans* →	No effect
<u>candidal vaginiasis</u> (rat) →	*C. albicans* →	↓ Candida in vaginal secretion
2. Therapeutic administration		
<u>Septicemia</u>		
Balb/c mice → $\Big\{$	*P. berghei* →	↑ Survival (circadian-dependent effect) < prophylactic regimen →No effect
	C. albicans ⟋ ID 100	→No effect
	⟍ ID 75	→Enhanced survival
<u>Chronic pyelonephritis</u> Balb/c mice →	*C. albicans*	↓ Candida colonization of the kidney, abcess formation and yeast urinary excretion
<u>Septicemia</u> Balb/c mice + cyclophosphamide	Methicillin-resistant *S. aureus*	Dose-dependent synergy with Ig + G-CSF
B) Sensitive pathogens		
<u>Septicemia</u>		
Balb/c mice Healthy Immuno- compromised (radiation, adriamycin) $\Big\}$	Enterobacteriaceae	↓ ED 50 (+++ IC mice) compared to Cefotaxime Cefoperazone Cefmenoxime Latamoxef
Balb/c mice Healthy IC $\Big\}$	Altered *K. pneumoniae*	↑ survival compared to cefotaxime

ID = Infective dose (pathogen): ID 100 → 100% deaths.

ED = Effective dose (antibiotics): ED 50 → dose that permits 50% survival.

Table 31 In Vivo IRM Activity of Cefodizime (models other than infection)

Model	Results
In vivo phagocytosis	
Sprague-Dawley rats	
CDZ before *H. influenzae* challenge	No bacteremia
Delayed-type hypersensitivity	
Balb/c mice—healthy	
CDZ one dose +	↑DTH (foot pad swelling test)
SRBC immunization	
Balb/c cortisone-treated (↓ DTH)	
same regimen as above	Restoration of DTH
Balb/c	
CDZ 7 doses	
oxazolone	No effect on DTH

Table 32 In Vitro IRM Activity of Cefodizime

Host defense effectors	Technique	Results
PMN (mouse, rats)	Cellular association	Binding-entry?
Macrophages (humans)	Cellular association	Binding-entry?

PMN } (healthy
Monocytes } humans)
	Phagocytosis
	Bactericidal function
		↑ non-opsonization
		  dependent
		↑ (co-operation with
		  O_2-independent systems)

	Chemotaxis, oxidative burst	No effect
PMN humans (diabetes mellitus)	Chemotaxis	Restoration
NK cells (healthy humans) IC (1 patient)	Lysis of target cells	No effect Restoration
Monocytes + LPS (± IFN ± T lymphocyte)	Cytokine	↓ TNF IL_1 production
Lymphocytes Molt-4 cells		Binding to membrane ↑ DNA synthesis ↑ DNA synthesizing enzyme activities
Splenic lymphocytes (NMRI mice)		↑ DNA synthesis
Bacterial virulence		

Synergy CDZ
  + complement
  + macrophages
	E. coli, S. marcescens,
	K. pneumoniae
		Effect superior to various
		  cephalosporins

Sensitive pathogens
  + CDZ
	K. pneumoniae, E. coli,
	S. aureus
		↑ Susceptibility to killing
		  via PMN, H_2O_2
		↑ Opsonization
		↑ Stimulation of
		  healthy/IC,
		  human/animal
		  phagocytes

Resistant pathogens	*P. aeruginosa*	↑ PMN stimulation +++ Not dependent on opsonization

IC = Immunocompromised.

Table 33 Ex Vivo IRM Activity of Cefodizime

Models	Results
1. Animals	
Balb/c mice—immunization SRBC (1 dose)	↑ B Ly responsiveness ↑ IgG production
Balb/c mice (7 doses)	No effect
NMRI mice (1 dose)	No effect
Balb/c mice	
T. gondii ⎫ ⎬ chronic infections *C. neoformans* ⎭	Restoration of the humoral response Restoration of IL-1, IFN production
Balb/c mice NMR I	↑ Oxidative activity of macrophage
2. Humans	
Healthy 4 g/day—6 days	↑ Phagocytosis (PMN, monocytes) (non-opsonization dependent)
Hemodialysis 5 x 2 g in 10 days	Restoration of blood leukocyte oxidative response
comparator: cotrimoxazole ⎱ placebo ⎰	No effect
Multiple myeloma 2 g/day—7 days	Restoration of monocyte chemotaxis (chrono-dependent effect)
Surgery 2 g/day—3 days (comparator: ceftriaxone)	↑ Phagocyte activity 24–72 h after last dose
Chronic bronchitis 4 g/day—6 days	↑ Phagocytosis
Elderly patients 2 g/day—8 days	↑ Phagocytosis
Lower respiratory tract infections 2 g/day—10 days	↑ Activity of a NK-cell subset ↑ CD4 lymphocytes
Anticancer chemotherapy 2 g/day—7 days	↑ T helper

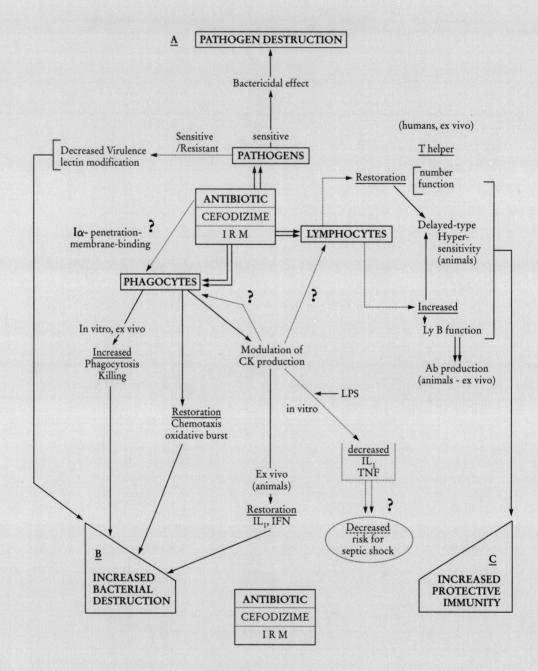

Figure 16 Cefodizime and infection.

BIBLIOGRAPHY

This book is the summary of more than 200 published papers. The most prominent reviews are listed below.

Phagocytes — Innate Immunity

Gabay J.E., Microbicidal mechanisms of phagocytes. Curr. Opin. Immunol. 1988; 1:36–40.

Gordon S., Keshav S., Chung L.P. Mononuclear phagocytes: Tissues distribution and functional heterogeneity. Curr. Opin. Immunol. 1988;1:26–53.

Haslett C., Savill J.S., Meahger L. The neutrophil. Curr. Opin. Immunol. 1989; 2:10–18.

Moncada S., Higgs E.A., Endogenous nitric oxide. Physiology, pathology and clinical relevance. Eur. J. Clin. Invest. 1991; 21:361–374.

Rappolee D.A., Werb Z. Secretory products of phagocytes. Curr. Opin. Immunol. 1988; 1:47–55.

Ross G.D., Complement and complement receptors. Curr. Opin. Immunol. 1989; 2:50–62.

Van Kessel K.P.M., Verhoef J. A view to a kill: Cytotoxic mechanisms of human polymorphonuclear leukocytes compared with monocytes and natural killer cells. Pathobiology 1990; 58:249–264.

Ziegler-Heitbrock H.W.L., The biology of the monocyte system. Eur. J. Cell. Biol. 1989; 49:1–12.

Specific Immune Responses

Born W.K. et al., The role of γδ T lymphocytes in infection. Curr. Opin Immunol. 1991; 3:455-459.

Cambier J., Lymphocyte subsets and activation. Curr. Opin. Immunol. 1988; 1:220–227.

Claman H.N., The biology of the immune response. JAMA 1987; 258:2834–2840.

Kaufmann S.H.E., Role of T cell subsets in bacterial infections. Curr. Opin. Immunol. 1991; 3:465–470.

Cytokines

Arai K. et al, Cytokines: Coordinators of immune and inflammatory responses. Annu. Rev. Biochem. 1990; 39:783–836.

Balkwill F., Cytokines–soluble factors in immune responses. Curr. Opin Immunol. 1988; 1:241–249.

Benton H.P., Cytokines and their receptors. Curr. Opin Cell Biol. 1991; 3:171–175.

Strober W., James S.P., The interleukins. Pediatr. Res. 1988; 24:549–557.

Microbial Virulence

Densen P., Mandell G.L., Phagocyte strategy versus microbial tactics. Rev. Infect. Dis. 1980; 2:817–838.

Kaufmann S.H.E., Reddehase M.J., Infection of phagocytic cells. Curr. Opin. Immunol. 1989; 2:43–49.

Spitznagel J.K., Microbial interactions with neutrophils. Rev. Infect. Dis. 1983; 5 (suppl. 4):S806–S822.

Immunodeficiencies

Buckley R.H., Immunodeficiency diseases. JAMA 1987; 258:2841–2850.

Figueroa J.E., Densen P., Infectious diseases associated with complement deficiencies. Clin. Microb. Rev. 1991; 4:359–395.

Graziano F.M., Bell C.L., The normal immune response and what can go wrong. Med. Clin. North Amer. 1985; 69:439–452.

Chronobiology

Levi F. et. al., When should the immune clock be reset? In: Temporal Control of Drug Delivery. Hrushesky W.J.M., Langer R., Theeuwes F., eds. Annals of the N.Y. Academy of Sciences, Vol. 618, 1991, pp. 312–329.

Antibacterial Agents and the Immune System

Anderson J.A., Franklin Adkinson N. Jr., Allergic reactions to drugs and biologic agents. JAMA 1987; 258:2891–2899.

Labro M.T., Immunomodulation by antibacterial agents: Is it clinically relevant? Drugs 1993; 45:319–328.

Mandell L.A., Effects of antimicrobial and antineoplastic drugs on the phagocytic and microbicidal function of the polymorphonuclear leukocyte. Rev. Infect. Dis. 1982; 4:683–697.

Sullivan T.J., Allergic reactions to antimicrobial agents: a review of reactions to drugs not in the β-lactam antibiotic class. J. Allerg. Clin. Immunol. 1984; 74:594–599.

Van den broek P.J., Antimicrobial drugs, micro-organisms and phagocytes. Rev. Infect. Dis. 1989; 11:213–145.

Cefodizime

Cefodizime Symposium. 17th International Congress of Chemotherapy, Berlin, June 1991.

Labro M.T., Cefodizime as a biological response modifier: A review of its in vivo, ex vivo and in vitro immunomodulatory properties. J. Antimicrob. Chemother. 1991; 26(supp. C):37–42.